CONTENTS

CHAPTER 3 | **WEEK 3 GOALS**   97

"For years I have been struggling with the right formula, the right attitude and the right protocol to follow to get [my health] to where I need to be. Dr. Gourmet proved to be the answer. With a healthy dose of 'get to exercising' and another dose of 'change your diet just a bit' I was well on my way. Within three months, six days a week of exercise and a redirect of my diet (no sodas, diet or otherwise, no fried foods, lots of vegetables and *only* red wine when I wanted to imbibe), I went from 172 pounds to my current weight of 157 pounds. And I feel terrific. The best part is bringing my pants to the tailor for alterations!"

—Mark R.

"My husband had a heart attack at age 54. He looked like the picture of health and we thought we were eating a healthy diet, so we were very surprised when this happened. I was searching for help when I stumbled upon [Dr. Timothy Harlan's] Dr. Gourmet website [and] recipes. What a relief! I was already stressed and this took such a load off knowing someone had already done the research. That was four years ago. My husband has lost 45 pounds since then, is very active and feels great too. Thank you Dr. Gourmet for the wonderful help!"

—Leah O.

"It has been wonderful experimenting with your recipes. . . . Your diet has allowed me to convert to healthy eating [and] continue to lose a pound a week. We are truly converted to your lifestyle . . . our pantry has changed, our recipes have changed . . . and friends and family have said that they feel they enjoy the food just for the flavor and the fact it is good for you is a bonus!"

—Julia G.

Design and production by Pauline Brown
Typeset in 11.5 point Adobe Garamond Pro by the Perseus Books Group

Library of Congress Cataloging-in-Publication Data

Harlan, Timothy S., 1958–
  Just tell me what to eat! : the delicious 6-week weight loss plan for the real world / Timothy Harlan.—1st Da Capo Press ed.
     p. cm.
  Includes bibliographical references and index.
  ISBN 978-0-7382-1452-8 (hardback)—ISBN 978-0-7382-1475-7 (e-book)
  1. Weight loss. 2. Cooking, Mediterranean. 3. Cookbooks. I. Title.
  RM222.2.H2434 2011
  613.2'5—dc22

                                                              2011002837

First Da Capo Press edition 2011

Published by Da Capo Press
A Member of the Perseus Books Group
www.dacapopress.com

Da Capo Press books are available at special discounts for bulk purchases in the U.S. by corporations, institutions, and other organizations. For more information, please contact the Special Markets Department at the Perseus Books Group, 2300 Chestnut Street, Suite 200, Philadelphia, PA 19103, or call (800) 810-4145, ext. 5000, or e-mail special.markets@perseusbooks.com.

10 9 8 7 6 5 4 3 2 1

JUST TELL ME WHAT TO EAT!

THE DELICIOUS 6-WEEK WEIGHT LOSS PLAN FOR THE REAL WORLD

Timothy S. Harlan, MD

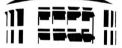

Da Capo
LIFE
LONG

A Member of the Perseus Books Group

When one undertakes any project of substance it is with the understanding that its completion relies on the aid and kindness of others. This book is no exception and its genesis lies in all my previous work and the many people who have helped shape the Dr. Gourmet message. To acknowledge everyone individually is impossible here, but know that I appreciate every one of you.

There are a few who are near and dear to this book. First and foremost are my patients, especially those who have contributed to this plan and my understanding of how food fits into their lives. Thanks to the entire Smith family, and especially Frank, BJ, and Barbara Jeanne Harlan. Cecilia Hatfield has my undying gratitude for her years of support and assistance. I so appreciate Kirsten Manges for her early work with me, and Ryan Fischer-Harbage for his expert guidance. Kathryn McHugh believed in this book. I am so grateful to her and everyone at Da Capo Press for helping shape this into the book you hold now (it is a much better book for those efforts).

My brother Bruce has believed from the very beginning and understood the importance of the Dr. Gourmet mission. Few people have the joy of working with their brothers that I have had in working with mine.

Morgan Ladd Harlan works every single day to make Dr. Gourmet a success. She is truly the jewel in my life but also a darn fine webmaster and editor and, most important, has a perfect palate. No one could hope for a better muse.

This book is for my mother Dr. Katherine B. Harlan, because my brother and I ask ourselves daily, "WWKD—What would Kate do?"

INTRODUCTION

It's no secret that obesity is the single most important issue facing us today. Sixty-five percent of Americans are overweight and 31 percent are obese, with the consequences including diabetes, high blood pressure, heart disease, strokes, and cancer. As a physician, when patients come to see me with these issues, it has been clear to me that they can treat their health problems with simple changes in their diet. Because I am also a chef, when I talk with them about eating healthier, they invariably say to me, "Tell me what to eat."

Like most doctors, I reply, "Well, cut down on fats and saturated fat and eat fewer calories. Eat more fruits and veggies." I show my patients lists of serving sizes of different foods. I tell them about Web sites where they could get information about eating healthy. We discuss the hype—and pitfalls—of popular fad diets. In short, I act like a doctor.

It was only after a patient said to me, for the third time, "No, no. Don't tell me about all that! Just tell me what to *eat*!" that I finally understood that I need to respond like a chef.

Christine was a young, newly married woman who was busy with her career and struggling with her weight. She was concerned about her mom's history of diabetes and her dad's heart disease, and wanted to lose weight. She had tried a variety of fad diets only to be repeatedly disappointed, and they had only served to confuse her. Christine literally wanted a prescription: exactly what to eat and when to eat it.

I realized that the chef in me could help her understand just what to eat, and the doctor in me could show her exactly what the research proves works best. I could easily write that prescription for her.

THE ISSUE

In spite of the issues people have with weight, I see patients sincerely wanting to make positive changes for themselves. Unfortunately, they encounter numerous, conflicting messages from media outlets reporting on the latest research, books touting the newest "revolutionary" diet, and weight-loss products that sound too good to be true and usually are. The media touts reliable information about nutrition every day, but it generally comes to us piecemeal, without context, without any useful discussion of whether it is of major or minor importance to health, and with no lasting advice on how to incorporate those findings into our daily lives. It's all well and good to talk about dietary fat, but how does this translate to your shopping cart? On the other hand, fad diets and highly touted weight-loss products come with simple instructions, usually based on pseudo-science that is at best questionable—and at worst, downright dangerous. The result is that such kooky diets have stolen real, delicious food from us. First, we couldn't have carbohydrates, and later, fats. This has just led to more confusion. Fiber's better, but wait a minute—it's all about a number, like the glycemic index. What has happened is that folks have ended up *not* focusing on what is most important—and that's the food.

Whenever I give health and nutrition lectures, people tell me about the diets they've tried and that eventually failed for them. Atkins, South Beach, Ornish, Zone, the blood type diet, detoxing, the cookie diet—I have heard it all and never had a patient truly succeed with them for the long term. Why? Fad diets don't help people really understand food. They never learn about how to make great-tasting food a part of their lives and how to plan, shop, cook, snack, and eat out. All they learn is a catchphrase based on dubious premises. So you stop eating carbs, but what happens when you get tired of not having delicious pasta? None of these diets help you understand what good food is; how to realistically maintain your weight loss; or how to plan, shop, and cook. What happens when you finish losing weight, using another silly idea, and don't know any more about how to eat healthy than when you started? The answer is that you gain all of the weight you lost (and usually more).

Further complicating the issue is that there's a disconnect between what we *want* to eat and what we tend to think of as healthy. The best research we have shows that diet is *the* key to living longer and living healthier, but it's very easy to hear about a new diet but get it wrong. If you hear Mediterranean diet you might think (as many of my patients do) that this means you'll be eating Greek salad and hummus. All of that conflicting and confusing information means there's something you may not know: that many of the foods you love are actually good for you!

The solution is not really a diet at all, but a reasonable, overall approach to eating delicious food and being healthy—and that's what this book gives you. It gives you your food back—real food, familiar food, and food that tastes great.

THE SOLUTION

I created weekly menus for Christine, all designed to fit into her schedule. Each recipe offered health, nutrition, and cooking information to instruct her in a digestible way, with step-by-step information, about the healthiest possible diet, one based on sound research. Because we do have great research on what works for a healthy diet and for weight loss, I was able to create a guide for her so that as she used the menus, she would learn exactly what works and why and also how to make it part of her life. As I shared it with more patients, the menu plan I created soon evolved, creating a prescription for "just what to eat." Patients told me time and again the recipes had to be recognizable foods that their family would eat, such as mac & cheese, shrimp enchiladas, and oven-fried chicken. "My family won't sit still for another kooky diet," was a common theme. These menus form the foundation for the 6-week program in this book. My plan is based on the simple premise that you *can* eat better, lose weight, and be healthier while still eating the foods you crave.

WHY ME? WHY DR. GOURMET?

I love food more than anyone you know. I say this often to my patients and when I lecture. People always laugh, but it's true. Ever since my first Peanuts cookbook (purchased at school at the age of eight), I have had a long love affair with cooking. My mom let me cook from the book and soon I could make potato dishes, bake cakes, and make my own taffy (pulling taffy as a nine-year-old was so very cool). I moved on to the *Joy of Cooking*, James Beard, Julia Child, and countless other books and chefs. My restaurant career began with washing dishes when I was eleven, and I owned my first restaurant at age twenty-two. I am truly happiest in the kitchen and love both cooking my old standby favorites and creating new recipes. After a couple of years as a chef-owner of a restaurant called Le Petite Café, I closed my restaurant to return to school to get a restaurant management degree. An illness in my family led me to medicine and eventually medical school. This was a revelation for me because I discovered just how strong the connection is between what we eat and how healthy we are. As I progressed in my training I was stunned to find the tremendous impact what we eat can have and that changes in diet have as profound an impact as almost any prescription medication on the market.

I wrote my first book on diet, *It's Heartly Fare*, when I was in medical school, and I've come light-years in my knowledge of food since then. This is partly because I have written and cooked constantly for twenty-five years, but it's also that during this time the scientific research on diet has shown us what works best. This 6-week plan you're holding in your hands is the culmination of my years of experience with cooking and health, based on the best evidence we have about diet, nutrition, and weight loss.

YOUR SECRET TO LONG-TERM
WEIGHT LOSS AND HEALTH FOR A LIFETIME

This is not the first book to offer a weight-loss plan. This is, however, a book that gives you a solution designed to actually fit into your life, one that you can thrive on *long-term*—helping you eat great food, lose weight, be healthier, live longer, and live better.

Just Tell Me What to Eat! is based on three simple principles.

#1. Eat the highest-quality calories that you can.

More than ever before, the research shows that if you want to lose weight, the most important thing to address is the number of calories you consume. However, that's not the only factor. The *quality* of the calories is key to getting the very most out of what you eat. For instance, lasagna made with less beef and more mushrooms has been shown to be more filling than one made with beef as the main ingredient, and you can save as many as 400 calories by eating the more satisfying recipe. More food, fewer calories, and delicious food is the principle behind Dr. Gourmet Quality Calories.

The recipes in this book have been carefully created to be low in overall calories but high in quality calories. Because they're delicious, it's easy for you to eat fewer calories and lose weight. The best part is that you don't have to think about it. There are six weeks of menu plans with simple, quick, tasty recipes, complete with shopping lists. By following the plan you'll learn everything you need about how to plan, shop, cook, and eat great, healthy food. I'll explain, step by step, why a recipe is better for you so that you can adapt your own favorites. When you are done with this plan you'll not be left hanging, as with a silly fad diet. You'll know and understand how you can keep eating the best-quality calories for sustained weight loss.

#2: Eat according to Mediterranean diet principles.

While the word "Mediterranean" might not seem like part of your world, this book translates those concepts into familiar recipes for you. There's tons of information about this starting on day 21, but for now understand that this simply means focusing on the nine principles of the Mediterranean diet and incorporating them into day-to-day life. By focusing on more vegetables, legumes, fruit and nuts, whole grains, seafood and great-quality oils alongside lean meats and quality dairy, favorite dishes are easily transformed. For instance, there's nothing more familiar than a good bowl of chili, and by using better oil, lean meat, lots of veggies, and red beans, the translation from Mediterranean diet to your table is simple (and delicious). But it doesn't stop there. The menus include dishes from many cuisines—comfort food, American, French, Southwestern, Asian, Caribbean, Italian, Spanish, and more.

#3. Whenever possible, you should make your own meals.

The more you create fresh food from scratch, the healthier you will be. I'll show you clear evidence during the next six weeks why making your own meals as often as possible is the key for your long-term success. This can be as simple as making a pot of soup on Sunday to taking a peanut butter and jelly sandwich to work. By cooking for yourself and your family, you'll get the best quality calories but also understand more of exactly what is in your food.

Virtually all diet books ask you to plow through pages and pages and pages of dense information explaining why you can't lose weight. Often that information is merely the authors' theories with no real supporting proof. Only after spending all that time reading do you get to eat—and then these plans often turn out to be odd collections of dishes and meal plans that most of us would never think of eating in the first place. I honestly don't believe that people crave hot tea and lemon with a handful of nuts for breakfast. Nor do they think, "Hmm, for dinner tonight I really want a plain piece of baked salmon." There's more to life than that!

When we're asked what we *want* to have for dinner, most of us think of real food, such as fettuccine Alfredo, hamburgers, fried chicken, and taco salad. A lot of times we simply don't want to think about dinner, preferring something out of the freezer, out of a package, or made by someone else in a restaurant. All of these real-world options are included in this book, laid out for you over a six-week meal plan that lets you mix and match real-world foods and eat what you know and love.

FOLLOWING THE PRESCRIPTION

It's rather simple, really. There are six weeks of meal plans and recipes to follow, along with shopping lists to help you plan. Every day during those six weeks you'll learn how to cook great food and about the real science behind healthy eating. But instead of having to read fifty thousand words before you ever get to eat a bite of food, you'll just read a little bit more of the prescription—the "nutrition rules"—each day. You'll find info marked Chef Tim Says . . . or Dr. Tim Says . . . to help you understand the best cooking techniques and state-of-the-art health information. By the end of six weeks you'll know what quality calories are, you will have lost weight, you'll know *why* you lost weight, and most important, you'll know how to keep it off and stay healthy going forward.

Again, the most important thing is that you must make your own meals. This is the key to success. *The more you create fresh food from scratch, the healthier you will be and the more you will learn.* For those inevitable times that you find yourself on the run, I've included options for a convenience meal (such as Lean Cuisine or Weight Watchers) or for eating in a restaurant, although I must say you're better off learning not to depend on these. Either way, what I want most is for you to *plan your meals* for the week on the Saturday before the week starts. Look at your schedule for the coming week, decide how much time you have for cooking on a particular day, and then choose the meal option that will suit your day the best.

The plan calls for you to cook four to six nights per week, using leftovers to make your life easier. For instance, in this plan, many days have recipes such as chili or beef stew that will leave enough to have leftovers later. If you know that the kids have soccer practice on Wednesday or that you have a late meeting scheduled, you might want to choose to eat out that night. Likewise, having your week planned is useful, but life doesn't always follow that plan. By having some basics in your pantry and freezer, you can use a Dr. Gourmet Pantry Meal recipe such as spaghetti with tomato sauce or tamale pie and you'll always have a healthy dinner no matter what comes your way.

During these weeks you will learn how to take stock of yourself, plan to act, and accomplish your goals. I also want you to read the information that is included with each day's meal plan and recipes. It's not a lot, but if you do this each day, at the end of two months' time you'll have a good understanding of why and how you can keep the weight off.

For the first four days, have only one serving of the given recipes for breakfast, lunch, and dinner. This will be less food than you are used to. If you are hungry between meals, have a piece of fruit or 100-calorie package of microwave popcorn. Starting on Day 5 you will find instructions for the number of calories personalized for you.

I recommend that you not drink alcohol until the day that it is discussed in the book. Alcohol is clearly a beneficial part of the Mediterranean diet (more about this, too), but early on in this plan it's best to just not have any, if for no other reason than because you don't need the extra calories.

Lastly, when you finish the six weeks, you should repeat the entire plan at least once, following the meal plans and reading the information again. After that, you'll have a solid understanding of what great and healthy food is all about. There are also tons of ongoing support at the Dr Gourmet.com Web site.

WHAT YOU CAN EXPECT

One of the biggest issues that I encounter with patients is their unrealistic expectations of weight loss. It's pretty typical for a forty-year-old to come to see me and I have to tell the individual that he or she is 40 pounds overweight. People are always motivated when they go see their doctor, and will almost always say something like, "No problem, Doc, I'm gonna lose this forty pounds in the next three months and I'll be fine."

This attitude is reinforced by hundreds of diet plans and thousands of pills that advertise, "LOSE 20 POUNDS IN TWO WEEKS!!!!!" They show marvelous before-and-after pictures of people who have lost weight. Think about this a minute. You're smart. You know as well as I do that it's a scam. Those before-and-after pictures are fake!

An increasing number of us each year are considered overweight and obese. Most of us might know one or two people who have successfully lost weight and kept it off—but that's it. It just doesn't often happen that people maintain their weight loss. Why?

One answer lies in people's expectations of how much and how fast they want to lose, compared to how much weight is actually healthy to lose over any period of time. When I tell you that 2 to 4 pounds a month is about right for healthy, sustained weight loss, that just is not what you want to hear. "LOSE 3 POUNDS IN FOUR WEEKS!!!!!" just doesn't have quite the sexy sales punch of the diet pill scams.

Sorry. Reality sucks sometimes.

That realistic weight loss does, however, have the ability to last for you and you can lose "20 POUNDS IN 26 WEEKS!!!!!" The best part is that when you do this the right way, with realistic expectations, you'll keep the weight off.

You should know up front that I am not going to spend a lot of time talking about every little hormonal response that happens when you eat. Such things as insulin response, leptin, and grehlin are not why our culture is overweight. I am sorry. It is not your genes. It's what's in your cupboard and refrigerator and what you put in your mouth. I am, however, going to tell you about the best-quality research that we have about what does work. What I want you to know is why you should eat better and lose weight and the best practices for how to do it.

We are told all our lives to excel, do more, "Reach for the stars." Losing weight and keeping it off for the long term doesn't work that way. Actually, if you will just relax and chill a bit, you'll succeed. Slow, steady, and delicious are the key. *Just Tell Me What to Eat!* presents a plan that wants you to do well and reach for the stars, but to do it consistently and for the long haul.

THE MEDITERRANEAN DIET IS THE DIABETIC DIET

A lot of folks who are overweight have diabetes or are at very high risk for developing diabetes. You might be one of those and might be asking whether this book can help you. It can!

Over the years there have been a number of different diet plans for diabetics. For a long time they were taught to use exchange lists. That method worked well, but was complicated and difficult to use. More recently the training has focused on counting carbohydrates at each meal or snack. For type 1 diabetics (those who take insulin), carefully regulating when and what they eat is vital, and counting carbs works well for them. The majority of diabetics, however, have type 2 diabetes and don't take insulin. This type is most often the result of being overweight or obese. I have long felt that simply following a healthy diet is the best choice for both types of diabetics.

In one of the lectures that I give medical students on nutrition, I cite multiple studies showing that diet can have as powerful an effect on controlling cholesterol as can medications. We know that a Mediterranean-style diet can help folks lose weight, prevent high blood pressure, and avoid diabetes. But can it also treat diabetes? A study published in the *Annals of Internal Medicine* says yes.[1] A resounding yes!

Researchers in Naples, Italy, randomized 215 type 2 diabetics to either a low-fat diet similar to the one recommended by the American Diabetic Association, or a Mediterranean-style diet providing about 50 percent of calories from carbohydrates and 30 percent from fat. These were patients who had hemoglobin A1c levels less than 11 percent (the A1c level is a measure of diabetic control of blood sugars, with good control being under 7 percent).

In both diets, calories were restricted to 1,500 per day for women and 1,800 per day for men. In the Mediterranean-style diet, 30 percent or more of the calories came from fat, with olive oil as the main source of added fat. The low-fat diet was based on American Diabetic Association guidelines, being rich in whole grains, with a restriction of additional fats, sweets, and high-fat snacks, and a target of less than 30 percent of calories from fat.

The study looked at the number of participants who needed to be put on medication for their diabetes. The researchers set the goal of having a hemoglobin A1c over 7 percent for more than three months as the criteria for starting medication. The results are pretty amazing. Those following the Mediterranean style diet avoided medication 56 percent of the time, while 70 percent of those following the low-fat American Heart Association–style diet ended up taking meds. Those on the Mediterranean-style diet also lost more weight and had a greater improvement in their cholesterol and blood pressure.

Until this research there has not been proof of just how powerful the Mediterranean diet can be for diabetics, but now, thankfully, we finally have the evidence we need. The principles, menus, and recipes in this book can definitely help you treat or prevent diabetes.

A NOTE ON EXERCISE

I want you to exercise almost as much as I want you to eat better. The research is clear about the importance of exercise for weight loss. In one large study,[2] the difference between those who were successful losing weight and those who did not lose weight was exercise. Over 46 percent of those who did lose weight exercised for thirty minutes or more each day. The same number reported adding physical activity to their daily routine as part of their strategy.

But you'll find my plan doesn't give you day-by-day information about how to work out. Why? Well, quite simply, that's not what I do for a living. I am a chef and a physician. While I do exercise regularly, I am not an expert. However, we have extensive exercise information and plans on the DrGourmet.com Web site to help you get started and stay motivated.

The good news is that it actually doesn't take much exercise to have a positive impact on your health. Thirty extra minutes per day is all you need—that's only two and a half hours each week! All it takes is simply *making the decision* that you are going to commit to exercising as part of your life and part of your plan—and then making the time for it.

The first part of your decision is choosing what to do.

Walking is the easiest way to start. It's an especially good choice if you haven't been exercising in a while, because you can start slowly. Start with twenty minutes per day and commit to walking as many days a week as possible. Every three days or so, add two minutes to your walk. Keep track of this along with your Food Diary (see Day 7). Work your way up to walking between thirty and forty minutes at a time.

The second step is to find other exercises that you love to do. Jog, swim, rollerblade, bicycle, aerobics, lift weights, Pilates . . . anything. It doesn't matter. As the Nike ad says, just do it. Mix it up. Walk two or three days a week, and other days, go to the gym or bicycle. You probably won't exercise every day, but that's okay. Schedule exercise for most days—five days per week is optimum. By committing to exercise as part of your life, you commit to living longer and living better.

WATER WORKS FOR WEIGHT LOSS!

For a long time there have been recommendations about water consumption, the most common being to drink eight glasses of water per day for optimum health. The best recommendation we have right now is to let thirst be your guide.

That said, many diets have included this instruction with the idea that filling up on water can help you lose weight. The interesting thing is that historically, there hasn't been good research about whether drinking water can help you lose weight. Until now . . .

Dr. Brenda Davy and her colleagues looked at forty-eight adults over the course of a twelve-week low-calorie diet plan. Half of the participants drank 16 ounces of water before each meal, while the other half did not. By the end of the study, the water drinkers had lost around 15½ pounds and the non–water drinkers only 11 pounds. The one caveat is that the folks in this study were between ages fifty-five and seventy-five. This is one of the longer and better designed studies, but previous smaller studies in younger age groups have had mixed results.

Even so, it's nice when things go from being an old wives' tale to solid, usable information. If you are working on losing weight, drinking water before each meal may actually be a powerful, proven tool that's cheap, easy, calorie free, natural, and good for you.

IT'S TIME TO EAT

I am really thrilled for you and your decision to improve your life and health. I wrote *Just Tell Me What to Eat!* to not only show you why you should eat better, but also exactly how you can do it. I recognize that you live in the real world and eat real food, so I have made this a practical plan that you can easily make part of your daily life. These principles are the ones that research has proven time and again to help you lose weight, live longer, live better, and best of all, eat great food!

CHAPTER 1 | *WEEK 1 GOALS*

Your first week is about learning the basics. I want you to get cooking right away, so the first day begins with one of my favorite meals, fettuccine Alfredo. You might not expect a recipe like fettuccine Alfredo in a diet plan, but this book is about both great food and about learning how to cook and eat to change your life, so we have to get some of the fundamentals out of the way.

The first three days begin with understanding the basic structure of a healthy breakfast, lunch, and dinner. I want you to keep these basics in mind throughout the following weeks, so it's a good idea to return to these three chapters again now and then to review them. They form the foundation of daily eating and will give you the framework to build your own menus.

The second half of the week is about taking stock of where you are and setting weight-loss goals for yourself: How much should you weigh and how much should you be eating to get there?

Just as important, you will need to set realistic targets for yourself. Getting to a healthy weight takes some time and starting out with an understanding of this is the first step to success. Likewise, keeping track of those goals and your progress is just as important.

Finally, in this first week, you'll learn a few key cooking techniques as well: how to make a white sauce, roasting, searing, and the best techniques for making pizza.

This week, you'll:

▌ Learn the fundamentals of a healthy breakfast, lunch, and dinner
▌ Assess your ideal weight and daily calorie intake
▌ Set your own goals
▌ Start keeping track of your progress

WEEK 1 | MENU

Throughout this plan I have provided menus and shopping lists for you. You should get in the habit of spending time once each week planning the upcoming seven days and assessing the previous week. Planning your meals is critical to eating well and eating healthy, and creating weekly menus and shopping lists are the building blocks of weekly planning. Having the right ingredients on hand to make these meals is another building block of eating healthy. (You'll learn more about creating menus on Day 18, but for now you can simply follow the plan.) This weekly planning time is also the time to consider your progress and reassess the goals that you will set for yourself on Days 4, 5, and 6.

Each week I'll show you your options for your dinner meal for each day of the week. You may choose to cook (which I hope you'll do the vast majority of the time), eat a convenience meal, or go to a restaurant. Look at your schedule for the upcoming week: Will you have time to cook or will you be too busy getting the kids to soccer or baseball? Or, perhaps you and your spouse like to go out to dinner once a week? Whatever you do, know what you're going to do beforehand so that you'll have the ingredients in the house.

A personalized shopping list for Week 1 can be found at DrGourmet.com/shoppinglist.

WEEK 1 MENU

RECIPE	CONVENIENCE FOOD ALTERNATIVE	RESTAURANT MEAL ALTERNATIVE
DAY 1		
Fettuccine Alfredo with Shrimp and Broccoli	Michael Angelo's Italian Natural Cuisine Chicken Alfredo with Broccoli	Panera Bread Tomato & Fresh Basil Crispani and Low-Fat Vegetarian Garden Vegetable Soup or Olive Garden Minestrone and Garden Salad
DAY 2		
Roasted Salmon and Corn Relish	Lean Cuisine Salmon with Basil or Lean Cuisine Lemon Pepper Fish	Red Lobster Garlic-Grilled Jumbo Shrimp or Red Lobster Grilled Fish
DAY 3		
Lentil Chili and Salad with Tomato-Chive Dressing	Health Valley Mild Black Bean Chili or Amy's Organic Low-Fat Medium Black Bean Chili	Wendy's Large Chili or Wendy's Spring Mix Salad
DAY 4		
Blackened Redfish, Dirty Rice, and Maple-Sweetened Collard Greens	Lean Cuisine Szechuan Style Stir Fry with Shrimp or Lean Cuisine Lemon Pepper Fish	P. F. Chang's Seared Ahi Tuna (sauce on the side) or P. F. Chang's Cantonese Scallops
DAY 5		
Leftover Lentil Chili and Salad with Tomato-Chive Dressing	Amy's Mexican Casserole or Amy's Tortilla Casserole	Ruby Tuesday Half-Serving Fresh Avocado Quesadilla with a Salad Bar (take other half for lunch tomorrow)
DAY 6		
Asian Peanut Chicken with Noodles	Lean Cuisine Chicken in Peanut Sauce or Kashi Sweet and Sour Chicken	Applebee's Tortilla Chicken Melt
DAY 7		
Barbecue Chicken Pizza	Kashi All Natural Mediterranean Pizza	Ruby Tuesday White Bean Chicken Chili

DAY 1 | *EAT WHOLE GRAINS WITH SOME PROTEIN AND FRUIT FOR BREAKFAST (AND DON'T SKIP BREAKFAST!)*

There are a lot of reasons to make breakfast the cornerstone of your new life. When you wake up in the morning, you've already gone for twelve to fourteen hours since eating dinner the night before. Skipping breakfast and waiting for a coffee break or until lunch before you eat adds even more time, so by the time you do eat, your body may have been without food for up to eighteen hours. What's worse is that when your coffee or lunch break does come around, you're hungry enough to eat with your stomach and not with your head. (You know just what I mean. Your tummy is hollering at you, "Hey, I am *hungry*! That doughnut looks good! Just one bite. Please!")

There is now a ton of research showing that extended periods of starvation does actually slow your body's metabolism: since there's not enough energy coming in, our body works to preserve the calories we have stored, making it harder to lose weight.

Studies show that people who usually skip breakfast tend to have a higher body mass index (BMI) than do those who regularly eat breakfast.[1] (BMI is a measure of weight in relation to height, which is used by researchers. More about this on Day 4.) Those breakfast eaters also tend to eat more regularly throughout the day; and smaller, regular meals are clearly associated with being more successful at controlling your weight. Eating breakfast also means you'll be less likely to eat between meals, and when you do, you're more likely to snack more responsibly.

We also know that *what* you eat every morning may be equally important to eating healthy and weight loss. In one study, those who ate cereals or bakery items for breakfast had a lower BMI than did people who ate meat and eggs,[2] but this could be because the meat and egg eaters simply ate more calories. Eating whole-grain or cooked cereals seemed to be better than ready-to-eat cereals or baked goods (possibly because of the higher fiber content). In fact, one study comparing whole-grain cereal, lower-fiber cereal, and white bread for breakfast showed that participants ate less at the next meal when they chose the food with the higher amount of fiber.[3]

Eating breakfast is good for your health in more ways than just weight control. Those who ate cereal for breakfast had a much lower risk of heart failure, in one study.[4] Another study showed that women who skipped breakfast had higher total cholesterol and LDL (bad) cholesterol than those who started the day right.[5]

I could easily go on, but you get the idea. Grandma was right (she knew it all along): Breakfast is the most important meal of the day. Begin your day with high-fiber cereals or whole-grain bakery goods, and you'll be less likely to snack throughout the day. Start your day right!

Here are some guidelines to help you choose a healthy breakfast. You'll use these guidelines to make your breakfast choices for the forty-two days of the program.

A breakfast "serving" should be built with a good-quality carbohydrate, a protein source, and some fat. It's a good idea to pair a fruit with your breakfast to provide good-quality calories and add fiber that will sustain you through the morning. For instance, a breakfast serving would be cereal (which is mostly carbohydrates) with milk (which is mostly protein with some fat). Another good example might be a slice of whole wheat toast (again, mostly carbohydrates) with an egg (mostly protein with some fat). Either of these, paired with a fruit selection, is a single serving. For the first week, you will have only one serving. In the weeks to come, you will determine the number of servings best tailored for you.

Weekday Breakfast Option No. 1

CEREAL WITH MILK (OR YOGURT) AND A PIECE OF FRUIT

Cereals should have about 100 to 150 calories in a serving. Choose higher-fiber and low-sugar cereals.

½ cup of skim or 1% milk on your cereal is ideal. Using ½ cup of nonfat yogurt is even better.

Weekday Breakfast Option No. 2

BREAD WITH TOPPING, A PROTEIN, AND A PIECE OF FRUIT

Breads should be consumed with a protein. Select one from the bread choices, one topping for your bread, and one choice from the protein list. Making muffins or quick breads on Saturday or Sunday is a great way to have a quick, delicious breakfast on hand throughout the week. It's healthier and you'll save a lot of money over that fast-food sausage biscuit.

Weekend Breakfast Options

On weekends you can eat the same breakfast as you do during the week, or try one of the weekend breakfast menus and recipes at the back of the book.

WEEKDAY BREAKFAST OPTIONS—CEREALS		
CEREAL	AMOUNT PER SERVING	COMMENT
Cheerios	1 cup (30 grams)	Multigrain is best!
Kellogg's All-Bran Bran Buds	½ cup (45 grams)	
Kellogg's All-Bran Extra Fiber	1 cup	
Kellogg's All-Bran Original	1 cup	
Bite Size Shredded Wheat	1 cup (52 grams)	Not frosted
Raisin Bran	1 cup	
Total Whole Grain	1 cup	
Total Raisin Bran	1 cup	
Kashi Cinnamon Harvest	1 cup	
Kashi GoLEAN	1 cup (53 grams)	
Oatmeal	¼ cup	(before cooking)
Cream of Wheat	¼ cup	(before cooking)

A word about Cereal Bars: Cereal bars are for emergencies only. Eating a granola bar for breakfast is not a good substitute for the right breakfast. Many of them have a lot of added calories (usually as sugar) and don't include the protein that you need to help keep you satisfied through the morning.

WEEKDAY BREAKFAST OPTIONS—BREADS

BREADS	AMOUNT	NOTES
Slice of whole wheat toast	1 slice	Choose whole-grain breads, the more fiber, the better.
Bagel	½ large bagel	Choose whole wheat bagels.
Whole wheat English muffin	1 whole muffin	
Muffin or quick bread from recipe in the back of the book	1 muffin or slice of quick bread	
Whole-grain frozen waffle	1 waffle	Kellogg's Nutri-grain are okay; Kashi is better with much more fiber.

TOPPINGS AND SPREADS FOR BREADS	AMOUNT	NOTES
CHOOSE ONE ONLY		
Take Control Light Spread	2 teaspoons	
Promise Buttery Spread Light	2 teaspoons	
Smart Balance Light Buttery Spread	2 teaspoons	
Preserves or jam	2 teaspoons	Lower-sugar versions can save you calories.
Reduced-fat cream cheese	2 teaspoons	The "light" cream cheese is best for spreading. I don't much like the fat-free version and use it mostly in baking.
Take Control Light Spread and syrup or honey	2 teaspoons spread and 1 tablespoon syrup or honey	Topping for pancakes or French toast only

PROTEIN	AMOUNT	NOTES
1 large egg	1 egg	Cook it in as little fat as possible.
Peanut butter	2 tablespoons	A much better choice than other spreads
Low-fat cheese	½ ounce	
2%, 1%, or skim milk	½ cup	
Nonfat yogurt	1 cup	Choose yogurt with no added sugar.

A VEGGIE-FILLED SANDWICH AND FRUIT

1 sandwich made with:

1 slice whole wheat bread (Yes, this means that 1 serving of this sandwich is what most people think of as ½ sandwich.)
1 ounce lean ham, turkey, or roast beef, *or* 1 ounce reduced-fat cheese
lettuce, tomato, green peppers, cucumbers, or other veggies of your
choice (as much as you want)
1 tablespoon reduced-fat mayonnaise *or* mustard

1 piece fruit (may use fruit for midmorning or midafternoon snack)

Chef Tim Says . . . Save Calories by Enhancing "Key Flavors"

Each dish has fundamental flavors that are critical to the final taste of the dish. Emphasizing these ingredients to enhance them, while looking for ways to reduce calories, is the secret to creating healthier recipes without compromising flavor.

A lot of recipes depend on rich ingredients for both flavor and texture, and fettuccine Alfredo is my favorite example of this. The key flavors are Parmesan cheese, garlic, and olive oil. The easiest way to reduce the amount of the rich ingredients, such as Parmesan or olive oil, is to always cook with the best-quality products.

Because fresh Parmigiano-Reggiano cheese has so much more flavor than the stuff in the green box, you need less of it to get bold flavor. The same holds true for using a fruity extra-virgin olive oil. These ingredients may be more expensive, but you'll use less of them.

Pay attention to *all* of your ingredients. Even though the garlic doesn't have many calories, buy the freshest garlic and store it in a cool place out of direct sunlight, to make the most flavorful dish. You can create a creamy texture in your sauce by using a lower-fat cheese, such as a semisoft goat cheese, along with 2% milk. The result is the same intense flavor and creamy feel of the higher-calorie version of the recipe with less fat and calories.

Fettuccine Alfredo with Shrimp and Broccoli

SERVINGS: 2 ▌ **SERVING SIZE:** 2 OUNCES PASTA, 4 OUNCES SHRIMP AND BROCCOLI WITH SAUCE ▌ THIS RECIPE CAN EASILY BE MULTIPLIED ▌ **COOKING TIME:** 30 MINUTES

3 cups broccoli florets

1 teaspoon extra-virgin olive oil

8 ounces shrimp, peeled and deveined

2 cloves garlic, minced

2 teaspoons all-purpose flour

¾ cup chilled 2% milk

1 ounce semisoft goat cheese or light cream cheese

1 ounce Parmigiano-Reggiano cheese, grated

4 ounces whole wheat fettuccine

NUTRITION FACTS

Serving size 2 ounces pasta
Servings 2
Calories 539
Calories from Fat 122
Total Fat 14 g (21%)
Saturated Fat 6 g (32%)
Trans Fat 0 g
Monounsaturated Fat 4 g
Cholesterol 194 mg (65%)
Sodium 547 mg (23%)
Total Carbohydrates 61 g (20%)
Dietary Fiber 8 g (34%)
Sugars 8 g
Protein 47 g
Vitamin A (26%)
Vitamin C (215%)
Calcium (47%)
Iron (35%)

*Parenthetical percentages refer to % Daily Value.

Rich, creamy sauces can be healthy. Start with less fat, cook the roux carefully, stir constantly when adding the liquid, and thicken with a lower-fat creamy cheese.

This is a quick weeknight meal that uses only two pans and cleans up easily. It's so rich and familiar that any family will love it. You can substitute almost any veggie that strikes your fancy; asparagus or zucchini are especially good choices.

1. Place 3 quarts of water in a large saucepan over high heat and bring to a boil. Add the broccoli florets and lower the heat until the water is simmering.

2. Cook for about 5 minutes. Using tongs, remove the florets and place them on a paper towel to drain. Leave the water in the saucepan.

3. While the broccoli is cooking, heat the olive oil in a 10-inch nonstick skillet over medium heat and add the shrimp. Cook for about 3 minutes on each side and transfer to a plate.

4. Add the minced garlic to the pan. Cook very slowly and stir frequently. Do not allow the garlic to brown or it will become bitter. Add the flour slowly and cook for about 1 minute. Stir continuously to blend the oil and flour. The mixture will be like coarse cornmeal. Cook gently so the mixture doesn't brown.

[CONTINUES]

> *Dr. Tim Says . . .*
> **Eat More Garlic**
>
> Garlic is good for you. Among the benefits: It tastes great, is low in calories (13 for three cloves), has essentially no fat or salt, no cholesterol, is pretty high in vitamin C, and has been shown to lower cholesterol at least a little.[6]

5. Slowly add the cold milk, whisking to keep the sauce from forming clumps. Blend in all of the milk until the sauce is smooth and begins to thicken. Add the goat cheese and whisk as it melts. When the sauce is smooth, add the Parmigiano-Reggiano and whisk as it melts until the sauce is creamy. Lower the heat to very low.

6. Add a couple of cups of water to the saucepan you cooked the broccoli in and heat the water to a boil. Add the fettuccine and cook until just tender (12 to 15 minutes for dried pasta).

7. When the pasta is almost done, add the shrimp and broccoli to the Alfredo sauce and toss to coat well. Increase the heat to medium.

8. Drain the pasta well and then add it to the sauce, tossing to coat thoroughly.

Day 1 Alternative Dinner Choices

CONVENIENCE MEALS

Michael Angelo's Italian Natural Cuisine Chicken Alfredo with Broccoli

RESTAURANT MEALS

Panera Bread Tomato & Fresh Basil Crispani and Low-Fat Vegetarian Garden Vegetable Soup or

Olive Garden Minestrone and Garden Salad

DAY 2 | *YOU MUST MAKE YOUR OWN LUNCH*

There's tons to be said for how much you can change your health (and your weight) by making your own lunch. Once again, research shows that skipping meals—breakfast or lunch (or both)—makes it harder to lose and maintain a healthy weight.

After talking with patients about breakfast, I ask them what they have for lunch. Most of them admit that they don't plan what they are going to eat and end up in fast-food joints or ordering take-out meals. Not many people take their lunch to work, yet making your own lunch is the best way to make sure you get the highest-quality calories. On this plan, it's important that you make your lunch every day and take it to work with you.

The easiest thing for most people to do is to make a sandwich. Following are some guidelines for items that you should pick up at the grocery store and keep on hand for making a quick and easy lunch. Making a sandwich takes no time at all and the calories you will save add up fast. A peanut butter and jelly sandwich with an apple is about 400 calories. That fried rice you might order from the Chinese takeout, however, is well over 700 calories. That 300-calorie savings every day represents about ½ pound per week of weight loss.

Just as important is all the money you'll save. Making a sandwich at home will cost you about $1. Eating out will average about $7. That's a savings of $30 per week or about $1,500 per year: enough for a pretty nice vacation.

Lunch Guidelines

As with breakfast, a lunch "serving" should be built with a good-quality carbohydrate, a protein source, and some fat. It's a good idea to pair fruit with your lunch as well. For instance, a lunch serving might be bread (mostly carbohydrates) with peanut butter (mostly protein with some fat) paired with a fruit selection. For the first week, you will have only one lunch serving each day. In the weeks to come, you will determine the number of servings best tailored for you.

SANDWICHES	

WHOLE SANDWICH (2 SERVINGS)
2 slices whole wheat bread with
  2 ounces lean meat or
  2 ounces reduced-fat cheese
	HALF SANDWICH (SINGLE SERVING)
	1 slice whole wheat bread with
	  1 ounce lean meat or
	  1 ounce reduced-fat cheese

SANDWICH FILLING CHOICES	
Lean ham slices	Reduced-fat Monterey Jack cheese
Lean turkey slices	Goat cheese
Reduced-fat Swiss cheese	2 tablespoons peanut butter

SANDWICH SPREADS AND TOPPINGS	
SPREADS	**TOPPINGS (AS MUCH AS YOU WANT)**
Hellman's or Best Foods Extra Light Mayonnaise: 1 tablespoon Any coarsely ground mustard: 1 tablespoon Dijon-style mustard: 1 tablespoon	Sliced tomato Lettuce Arugula (rocket) Mâche Spinach

SALADS

A lot of patients ask me about having a salad at lunch. This is a great idea! Most greens and veggies don't add up to many calories, and they are chock-full of fiber, vitamins, and antioxidants. Have a salad on its own or, better yet, choose the salad and half-sandwich combo.

Some dressings are included throughout this book. These generally have about 50 calories in a serving (avoid dressings that have more than 50 calories per serving). Remember to measure your dressing portion, and that if the greens are very dry, you will need less dressing—it will cling to the salad better.

LEFTOVERS FROM DINNER

Dinner leftovers make the perfect lunch. It's a great idea to make extra the night before so you have something to take for lunch the next day. The rule of thumb is that a lunch serving is half of a dinner serving. Alternatively, 2 lunch servings = 1 dinner serving. For instance, if you made extra Salmon and Corn Relish today, you could take the leftover dinner serving as two lunch servings (remember, in the first week you are allowed two lunch servings, but once you have your plan tailored to you, as you will later, you may need more breakfast and lunch servings).

Roasted Salmon and Corn Relish

SERVINGS: 2 ▌ SERVING SIZE: 1 (4-OUNCE) SALMON FILLET WITH RELISH ▌ THIS RECIPE
CAN EASILY BE MULTIPLIED ▌ COOKING TIME: 30 MINUTES ▌ THE RELISH AND SAUCE
CAN BE MADE UP TO 24 HOURS IN ADVANCE. REHEAT GENTLY WHILE THE SALMON IS
ROASTING.

RELISH
1 red bell pepper
1 green onion, sliced
½ teaspoon grapeseed oil
1 cup (~1 ear) fresh corn
    kernels (frozen are
    okay)
1 tablespoon minced shallot
    (~1 small shallot)
1 small clove garlic, minced
1½ teaspoons fresh thyme,
    or ½ teaspoon dried
2 tablespoons dry white
    wine
1½ teaspoons freshly
    squeezed lime juice
1½ teaspoons honey
⅛ teaspoon salt
1 tablespoon minced fresh
    parsley

SAUCE
1½ teaspoons grapeseed oil
1 tablespoon freshly
    squeezed lime juice
1½ teaspoons honey
1½ teaspoons paprika
⅛ teaspoon salt

FISH
2 (4-ounce) salmon fillets
1 tablespoon chopped fresh
    cilantro

This recipe makes great leftovers. I like to make sandwiches from the salmon and relish but both go well chilled on top of salads.

People often think of vegetables as a side dish, but making them part of the whole meal is a great way to eat well and eat healthy. When you make the relish full of veggies to go with the salmon, you create a dish that stands on its own but has all the right elements—protein, carbohydrates, healthy fats—and is full of veggies (and flavor).

1. Preheat the oven to broil. Place the pepper in the oven and char, turning about every 3 minutes until black on all sides. Remove and place in a paper bag.

2. After 10 to 20 minutes, remove the pepper from the bag. Peel, seed, and set aside half of the pepper in the refrigerator for another recipe (put it on your sandwich!). Cut the remaining pepper half into ½-inch pieces. Slice the white part of the green onion separate from the green tops.

3. Heat the grapeseed oil in a heavy, large nonstick skillet over medium-high heat. Add the corn, the white part of the green onions, the shallot, and the garlic. Sauté gently until the corn begins to brown. Add the thyme and white wine. Cook over low heat until the wine evaporates.

[CONTINUES]

NUTRITION FACTS

Serving size 4 ounces salmon
   with relish
Servings 2
Calories 378
Calories from Fat 139
Total Fat 16 g (24%)
Saturated Fat 2 g (12%)
Trans Fat 0 g
Monounsaturated Fat 6 g
Cholesterol 70 mg (23%)
Sodium 362 mg (15%)
Total Carbohydrates 33 g (11%)
Dietary Fiber 5 g (19%)
Sugars 15 g
Protein 28 g
Vitamin A (82%)
Vitamin C (286%)
Calcium (4%)
Iron (12%)

*Parenthetical percentages
refer to % Daily Value.

4. Stir in the chopped bell pepper, lime juice, honey, salt, the green tops of the green onions, and the parsley. Remove from the heat.

5. Make the sauce: Stir together the grapeseed oil, lime juice, honey, paprika, and salt.

6. When almost ready to serve, preheat the oven to 400°F. Line a roasting pan or ovenproof skillet with foil. Place the salmon in the middle and top with the sauce. Place in the hot oven and roast for about 10 minutes.

7. While the salmon is roasting, gently reheat half of the corn relish.

8. Remove the salmon from the oven and place on plates. Top each fillet with one-quarter of the relish and garnish with fresh cilantro.

Chef Tim Says . . . Roasting Adds Flavor

Roasting is a cooking method that uses dry heat. The food is cooked at a high heat, often producing a browned, crispy surface and sealing in natural juices. The great thing about roasting is that you don't need added fat (and thus added calories). In this recipe and others that employ roasting, however, I also use a sauce to add flavor and some moisture.

Generally, use more tender pieces of meat, fish, or poultry for roasting. The pan should be large enough that the moisture that does escape from the food evaporates quickly, otherwise the steam will keep the food from browning properly. When roasting vegetables, it is important to use a large pan so that they do not touch one another. I try to leave at least one-quarter of the bottom of the pan exposed and stir the vegetables often.

Dr. Tim Says . . . Eat Fish and Reduce Your Risk of Heart Disease

Fish are some of the highest-quality calories we can eat. Numerous studies have shown that for both men and women, eating fish reduces one's risk of fatal heart attacks.[7] One study shows that just eating fish about once a week reduces the risk of fatal heart attack by at least a third, and consuming it more often reduces the risk even more: Those who eat fish two to four times per week cut their risk by over 40 percent.

The results were the same even when the study participants also ate other foods that might also have an effect on their risk of heart disease, such as fiber, eating more or less red meat and fruits and vegetables, or following a lower-saturated-fat diet.

Fish are a good source of protein, a great source of omega-3 fats (more on those later, on page 77), and low in calories (the perfect combo).

Day 2 Alternative Dinner Choices

CONVENIENCE MEALS

Lean Cuisine Salmon with Basil or
Lean Cuisine Lemon Pepper Fish

RESTAURANT MEALS

Red Lobster Garlic-Grilled Jumbo Shrimp or
Red Lobster Grilled Fish

DAY 3 | *ARRANGE YOUR DINNER PLATE*

One problem many people have is that they don't know what to actually put on their dinner plate. When I was growing up, we had the typical diner Blue Plate Special of "a meat and two veg." This isn't too far from what makes sense for a healthy dinner. But contributing to the problem is that the serving sizes at most restaurants have become much more than a single serving. This has carried over into people's dinner table at home, and so portions at home have gone from big to bigger to huge. So when you're considering dinner ideas, think also in terms of right-sizing your meal.

Let's say your dinner plate includes a protein, carbs, and a vegetable. A complete dinner should total about 500 calories.

Begin with the main course. By that I mean the protein you will have: fish, lean meat, shellfish, chicken, turkey, lamb, and so on. The rule of thumb for a single serving for an adult is *4 ounces* by weight. When you are reading recipes, keep this in mind, because many call for single-serving sizes of double or even triple this amount. With a 4-ounce serving coming in at around 150 to 200 calories, it's easy to see how in today's world folks can easily get too many calories.

That's why I'm a believer in weighing ingredients, especially when you are learning how to eat healthier. Knowing just what that 4 ounces looks like is important, and by weighing your food you'll learn exactly what a portion should look like.

STARCHES

GREAT STARCH/ CARB CHOICES	SINGLE SERVING SIZE	APPROXIMATE CALORIES (PER SERVING)
Whole wheat bread	2 slices	150
Whole wheat pasta	2 ounces	175
Potatoes	8 ounces	175
Yams	6 ounces	160
Brown rice	¼ cup (raw)	170
Wild rice	¼ cup (raw)	140
White rice	¼ cup (raw)	170
Corn (Yes, corn is a starch, not a vegetable.)	1 cup kernels	135
Couscous	¼ cup (raw)	160
Lentils	¼ cup (raw)	170
Beans	¼ cup (raw)	155

Once you've decided what you're having for the main course, it's time to think about the carbs. Combining protein with carbohydrates helps you feel satisfied for longer after a meal. There are lots of choices here, and a serving generally works out to somewhere between 150 and 250 calories. Keep in mind that making the higher-fiber choice such as brown rice, whole wheat pasta, and yams will be the best-quality calories.

Adding up the number of calories we have so far gets us to somewhere between 300 and 450 calories for the meal. That can be a bit of a wide mark, but for the most part it'll balance out over the long haul.

So that leaves the veggies. Quite simply, eat what you want. If you like carrots, cool. Peas? Perfect. Salad greens, peppers, onions, squash (in all its variations), cabbage—take your pick. Most are so low in calories that you can eat all you want, with some being as little as 25 calories up to as much as 100 in 4 ounces. At the same time, veggies are full of vitamins, antioxidants, and other healthy nutrients (more about this on Day 23).

Altogether, this will add up to between 325 and 550 calories for the whole meal (from the lowest combination to the highest).

Note that dinner doesn't always have to be a meat, starch, and veggie on your plate as you might get at the diner. The menu for today is a good example. There are plenty of veggies in the chili, and the lentils provide mostly starch but also some protein. The rest of the protein comes from the cheese, and there are even more veggies in the side salad.

It's a great idea to keep ingredients on hand for salads. If you keep lettuce, carrots, celery, peppers, cucumber, and the like on hand, you will always be able to get the extra servings of veggies that are so important to your health as well as to controlling your weight. Fixings for a side salad are especially important because they can help round out your dinner on those days when you have a convenience meal.

DAY 3 | DINNER

LENTIL CHILI AND SALAD WITH TOMATO-CHIVE DRESSING

> ### Dr. Tim Says . . . Eat Lentils
>
> Lentils are some of the highest-quality calories you can get. They are mostly carbs and are a member of the legume family, as are peas, peanuts, and beans. Along with those carbs, they have great-quality protein, are full of fiber to help lower cholesterol, and have tons of vitamins and minerals. Legumes are filling, and there is excellent evidence that eating only a single serving of them (e.g., lentils or chickpeas) each week lowers your risk of heart disease.[8] The best part? The more you eat, the lower the risk. Eating legumes four or more times per week reduces the risk of heart disease by as much as 22 percent.

Lentil Chili

SERVINGS: 4 ▌ **SERVING SIZE:** ABOUT 1½ CUPS ▌ THIS RECIPE CAN EASILY BE MULTI-PLIED ▌ **COOKING TIME:** 75 MINUTES

Save the leftover Lentil Chili and Tomato-Chive Dressing for dinner on Day 5.

1 tablespoon olive oil
2 cloves garlic, sliced
1 large onion, diced
1 (15-ounce) can no-salt-added crushed tomatoes
1 tablespoon chili powder
2 teaspoons ground cumin
1 teaspoon dried oregano
½ chipotle in adobo (optional)
¼ teaspoon salt
Freshly ground black pepper
1 cup dried lentils
6 tablespoons nonfat sour cream
6 ounces reduced-fat Monterey Jack cheese, shredded

NUTRITION FACTS

Serving size 1½ cups
Servings 4
Calories 386
Calories from Fat 106
Total Fat 12 g (18%)
Saturated Fat 6 g (32%)
Trans Fat 0 g
Monounsaturated Fat 4 g
Cholesterol 29 mg (10%)
Sodium 437 mg (18%)
Total Carbohydrates 44 g (15%)
Dietary Fiber 18 g (71%)
Sugars 8 g
Protein 27 g
Vitamin A (23%)
Vitamin C (34%)
Calcium (43%)
Iron (35%)

*Parenthetical percentages refer to % Daily Value.

This recipe makes great leftovers.

This is a fine chili that's a snap to make and full of flavor. It has it all: low calories, low fat, high fiber, garlic, cheese, sour cream—all the great things in life. If spicy foods give you heartburn, you should be fine if you leave out the chipotle pepper, as there's not much cumin or chili powder in each serving. If you like your chili spicy and don't have access to chipotle peppers, use cayenne, adding ⅛ teaspoon at a time to your preferred level of spiciness.

1. Place the olive oil in a large saucepan, over medium heat. Add the garlic and onion and cook, stirring frequently, until the onion has softened. Add the crushed tomatoes, chili powder, cumin, oregano, chipotle (if using), salt, and pepper to taste, and stir well.

2. Add 5 cups of water and the lentils and stir well. Lower the heat to medium-low and simmer until the lentils are cooked through but not mushy, 45 minutes to an hour.

3. Serve topped with 1½ tablespoons of sour cream and 1½ ounces of Monterey Jack cheese per serving.

Salad with Tomato-Chive Dressing

SERVINGS: 6 ▌ **SERVING SIZE:** ¼ CUP DRESSING ▌ THIS RECIPE CAN EASILY BE DOUBLED

1 (5-ounce) can low-sodium V8 juice
1 tablespoon extra-virgin olive oil
2 tablespoons tomato paste
2 tablespoons coarsely ground Dijon mustard
2 tablespoons red wine vinegar
1 tablespoon pure maple syrup
¼ teaspoon salt
2 tablespoons chives, chopped
2 cloves garlic, minced
Lettuce, tomatoes, mushrooms, peppers, and so on

NUTRITION FACTS

Serving size ¼ cup dressing only
Servings 6
Calories 44
Calories from Fat 22
Total Fat 3 g (4%)
Saturated Fat 0.5 g (2%)
Trans Fat 0 g
Monounsaturated Fat 2 g
Cholesterol 0 mg (0%)
Sodium 214 mg (9%)
Total Carbohydrates 5 g (2%)
Dietary Fiber 1 g (2%)
Sugars 4 g
Protein 1 g
Vitamin A (10%)
Vitamin C (14%)
Calcium (1%)
Iron (2%)

*Parenthetical percentages refer to % Daily Value.

This is a simple and very fresh-tasting dressing from ingredients you might already have around the house. Pair it with some lettuce, tomato, carrots, mushrooms, peppers, and so on, for a great side salad that'll come in under 100 calories.

I based this dressing on one my mother made when I was growing up. She called this "French dressing" and made it with some of the same ingredients. I added the chopped chives to give it a fresh summer flavor.

This dressing will keep well for about a week in the fridge.

Place all the dressing ingredients in a shaker bottle and shake vigorously. Chill for at least 2 hours before serving on the salad.

Chef Tim Says . . .
Dry Those Salad Greens
Make sure that your salad greens are dry, dry, dry before tossing the dressing with them. If they are damp, the dressing won't stick as well and you will have to use more. Usually 2 tablespoons of a well-made dressing (one that is well blended) is enough if the greens are dry. To dry lettuce, use a salad spinner— a must-have in any kitchen.

CONVENIENCE MEALS

Health Valley Mild Black Bean Chili or
Amy's Organic Low-Fat Medium Black Bean Chili

RESTAURANT MEALS

Wendy's Large Chili or
Wendy's Spring Mix Salad

DAY 4 | *HOW MUCH SHOULD YOU REALLY WEIGH?*

Almost every day, patients ask me what they should weigh and how much weight they need to lose. I admit that sometimes I am a bit evasive—I'll say things like, "Start working on your weight, and I'll tell you when to stop."

Why aren't I more direct? Because people can be pretty unrealistic about their health and their weight. Usually people are shocked when I tell them what an ideal weight would be for them. "I haven't weighed that little since high school!" is a common response. The interesting thing is that for most of us, what we weighed in high school is close to what our ideal body weight should be. It's important information to know, first and foremost, so you have a healthy target, but also to help you know how many calories you should be eating to reach your goal weight.

There are a few ways to estimate what your best weight should be. Body mass index (BMI) is one of the most reliable guides for what a healthy weight is for you.

BMI is a rough estimate of body fat. The limitation is that it doesn't measure body fat directly, so the index can be misleading for those who have an especially high ratio of lean muscle mass to their overall weight. For the vast majority of us, however, BMI is a good indication of whether your weight is in a normal range for your height.

You no doubt already know that being overweight can have serious effects on your health. Being overweight and obesity have been linked to many illnesses, with heart disease, diabetes, high blood pressure, breast cancer, colon cancer, arthritis, and stroke being the most common problems.

I like to talk with my patients about the real consequences for them of these conditions. If your weight leads to having diabetes or a heart attack, will you be able to dance at your son's wedding? Will you live to see your daughter's first child graduate from high school? There's also real pain in simply carrying around too much weight: Arthritis of the knees, difficulty breathing, swelling of the ankles, and diabetic foot problems are just some of the facts of life for most people with a BMI in the obese range.

This table shows the range of weights for a *normal* body mass index. Simply find your height in inches in the left-hand column, then read across the row to find the number closest to your current weight. The number in the top of the column would then be your approximate BMI. A normal weight will fall between the weights for a BMI of 19 to 25. The ideal body weight for you is a BMI between 22 and 23.

NORMAL BODY MASS INDEX (BMI)							
BMI	19	20	21	22	23	24	25
HEIGHT INCHES	BODY WEIGHT POUNDS						
58	91	96	100	105	110	115	119
59	94	99	104	109	114	119	124
60	97	102	107	112	118	123	128
61	100	106	111	116	122	127	132
62	104	109	115	120	126	131	136
63	107	113	118	124	130	135	141
64	110	116	122	128	134	140	145
65	114	120	126	132	138	144	150
66	118	124	130	136	142	148	155
67	121	127	134	140	146	153	159
68	125	131	138	144	151	158	164
69	128	135	142	149	155	162	169
70	132	139	146	153	160	167	174
71	136	143	150	157	165	172	179
72	140	147	154	162	169	177	184
73	144	151	159	166	174	182	189
74	148	155	163	171	179	186	194
75	152	160	168	176	184	192	200
76	156	164	172	180	189	197	205

OVERWEIGHT/OBESE BODY MASS INDEX (BMI)

BMI	26	27	28	29	30	31	32	33	34	35
HEIGHT INCHES	BODY WEIGHT POUNDS									
58	124	129	134	138	143	148	153	158	162	167
59	128	133	138	143	148	153	158	163	168	173
60	133	138	143	148	153	158	163	168	174	179
61	137	143	148	153	158	164	169	174	180	185
62	142	147	153	158	164	169	175	180	186	191
63	142	147	153	158	164	169	175	180	186	191
64	146	152	158	163	169	175	180	186	191	197
65	151	157	163	169	174	180	186	192	197	204
66	156	162	168	174	180	186	192	198	204	210
67	166	172	178	185	191	198	204	211	217	223
68	171	177	184	190	197	203	210	216	223	230
69	176	182	189	196	203	209	216	223	230	236
70	181	188	195	202	209	216	222	229	236	243
71	186	193	200	208	215	222	229	236	243	250
72	191	199	206	213	221	228	235	242	250	258
73	197	204	212	219	227	235	242	250	257	265
74	202	210	218	225	233	241	249	256	264	272
75	208	216	224	232	240	248	256	264	272	279
76	213	221	230	238	246	254	263	271	279	287

For instance, if you are 63 inches tall (5 feet 3 inches), a good range for a healthy weight, whether you are male or female, is between 107 and 141 pounds.

WORLD HEALTH ORGANIZATION CLASSIFICATION

BODY MASS INDEX (BMI)	WORLD HEALTH ORGANIZATION CLASSIFICATION
Less than 18.5	underweight
18.5 to 24.9	normal weight
25 to 29.9	overweight
30 or more	obese
Greater than 35	very obese

Next, measure your waist-to-hip ratio. The waist-to-hip ratio (WHR) is calculated by dividing the measurement around your waist at the belly button by the measurement around your hips at the widest point.

The goal for men is a waist measurement of less than 40 inches and a WHR less than 0.9. For women, the goal measure is a waist under 36 inches and a WHR less than 0.8. Those with a WHR greater than 1.0 have been shown to be at much higher risk for heart disease and other health problems.

Researchers have labeled a high WHR the "apple" shape or "apple obesity." Studies have clearly shown that a high WHR is a very accurate predictor of illness. I generally discuss both WHR and BMI with my patients. (Note that it is possible to have a BMI in the overweight or obese range but still be healthy. For instance, Arnold Schwarzenegger at his fittest had a high BMI, but this was lean, muscular body mass and not fat.)

Now, for some of you, finding out your ideal weight and where you fall in the BMI chart is going to be shocking information. If you are overweight or obese, don't worry! You *can* get to a healthy weight. It takes some planning and work at taking action, but as you read through this book, each day you'll learn a little more about how to make that happen.

You've already made small changes that will make a big difference over time. As I mentioned on Day 2, making your own lunch is the *single easiest way to cut calories*. Save your money and save your life! Start making your lunch each day and taking it with you. It takes all of ten minutes to make a sandwich and put it in a bag with a piece of fruit. This is a critical part of this program. By making your lunch, you not only save money but you are in complete control of the amount of calories you'll have each day at that meal.

DAY 4 | DINNER

BLACKENED REDFISH, DIRTY RICE, AND MAPLE-SWEETENED COLLARD GREENS

Blackened Redfish

SERVINGS: 4 ▌ **SERVING SIZE:** 4 OUNCES FISH ▌ THIS RECIPE CAN EASILY BE MULTIPLIED, BUT YOU MUST USE A LARGE PAN ▌ **COOKING TIME:** 30 MINUTES

2 teaspoons paprika
1 teaspoon salt
¼ teaspoon onion powder
¼ teaspoon garlic powder
¼ teaspoon cayenne
¼ teaspoon freshly ground black pepper
¼ teaspoon dried thyme
¼ teaspoon dried oregano
4 (4-ounce) fresh red snapper fillets
Spray olive or grapeseed oil

NUTRITION FACTS

Serving size 4 ounces fish
Servings 4
Calories 121
Calories from Fat 15
Total Fat 2 g (3%)
Saturated Fat 0.5 g (2%)
Trans Fat 0 g
Monounsaturated Fat 0 g
Cholesterol 42 mg (14%)
Sodium 655 mg (27%)
Total Carbohydrates 1 g (<1%)
Dietary Fiber 1 g (4%)
Sugars 0 g
Protein 24 g
Vitamin A (14%)
Vitamin C (5%)
Calcium (4%)
Iron (3%)

*Parenthetical percentages refer to % Daily Value.

This recipe is so quick and simple, and there's nothing better than the taste of New Orleans. Using a cast-iron skillet will let you heat the pan until it is smoking hot, and that's key to the blackened spice crust. If you don't have an iron skillet, use a stainless-steel or aluminum pan, but not one coated with nonstick material.

Serve with Dirty Rice and Maple-Sweetened Collard Greens (recipes follow). The blackened redfish makes great sandwiches as leftovers.

1. Preheat the oven to 400°F. Place a large cast-iron skillet in the oven.

2. Combine the paprika, salt, onion powder, garlic powder, cayenne, black pepper, thyme, and oregano in a small bowl. Mix together until well blended.

3. When the pan is hot, place the fish on a cutting board, skin side down. Spray the fish lightly with oil and carefully dust the top of the fillets with the spice mixture.

4. Place the fish in the hot pan, skin side up, and return the pan to the oven. Cook for 8 to 10 minutes and serve.

Chef Tim Says . . . Use a Cast-Iron Skillet

Okay, you don't *have* to use a cast-iron skillet for this recipe, but it works great because it helps foods sear so well. Whether you use an iron skillet or not, the key to proper searing is a hot pan. This allows the food to cook quickly and to brown. It's important to not overcrowd the pan, or the moisture that comes from the food won't evaporate and your dish will steam instead. Overcrowding also lowers the temperature of the pan and you won't get that nice brown seared crust.

When you buy a cast-iron pan, you need to cure it to keep food from sticking. Here's how:

1. Place about 4 tablespoons of oil in the bottom of the pan and put the pan in an oven that has been preheated to 400°F. Use an oil without much flavor, such as canola.
2. After about 3 minutes, lower the temperature to 300°F and leave the pan in the oven for 45 minutes.
3. Turn off the oven and let the pan cool inside the oven.
4. When the pan is cool enough to touch, wipe out the excess oil with a paper towel.

Do not use detergent to clean a porous skillet, because soaps strip the oils (and thus your "cure") from the pan. Simply rinse the pan with hot water and wipe clean. To remove food that is stuck to the pan, scrub gently with salt or a plastic scrub pad.

Dr. Tim Says . . . Eat Brown Rice More Often

There is no doubt that brown rice is a healthier choice. Making the switch to brown rice can reduce your risk of getting diabetes. Switching from white rice to brown for just one serving per day has a significant lowering effect on your risk of developing diabetes, in fact, and this is likely because of the higher fiber content. Most folks aren't used to eating brown rice, however. One good way to make the transition can be to start by using instant brown rice products. They cook quickly, have all the fiber and nutrients of brown rice, and use varieties that are light and fluffy.

Chef Tim Says . . . Eat Rice

Rices are classified as either short, medium, or long grain. Long-grain rices are of the subspecies *indica*, while the shorter are *japonica*.

Long-grain rice is about four to five times as long as it is wide and has lighter, fluffier grains that separate when cooked. Because the starch content is lower, the rice doesn't stick together as easily as medium- or short-grain rice does. Basmati and jasmine rice are examples of long-grain rices. Both have light, aromatic flavors.

Short-grain rice is slightly rounded and plump. Its higher starch content makes for a creamy rice, and when cooked, the grains tend to stick together. Rice for sushi is made from short-grain rice. Arborio rice, a short-grain rice with a very high starch content, is the basis for Italian risotto as well as Spanish paella.

Dirty Rice

SERVINGS: 2 ▌ **SERVING SIZE:** ¾ CUP ▌ THIS RECIPE CAN EASILY BE MULTIPLIED ▌
COOKING TIME: 45 MINUTES

¼ teaspoon salt
½ cup uncooked brown rice
2 teaspoons olive oil
1 large shallot, minced
Green onions, sliced
    crosswise into white
    and green parts
¼ large green bell pepper,
    seeded and diced
¼ large red bell pepper,
    seeded and diced
¼ teaspoon ground cumin
½ teaspoon chili powder
½ teaspoon dried oregano
Cayenne

NUTRITION FACTS

Serving size about ¾ cup
Servings 2
Calories 244
Calories from Fat 55
Total Fat 6 g (10%)
Saturated Fat 1 g (5%)
Trans Fat 0 g
Monounsaturated Fat 4 g
Cholesterol 0 mg (0%)
Sodium 307 mg (13%)
Total Carbohydrates 43 g (14%)
Dietary Fiber 4 g (17%)
Sugars 4 g
Protein 5 g
Vitamin A (39%)
Vitamin C (154%)
Calcium (4%)
Iron (10%)

*Parenthetical percentages
refer to % Daily Value.

Brown rice is a perfect choice for this spicy rice recipe. The nutty taste of the brown rice helps balance the spicy flavor and more than doubles the fiber of using white rice.

1. In a medium-size saucepan, heat 2½ cups of water and the salt. When the liquid comes to a boil, stir in the brown rice.

2. Lower the heat to medium-low and simmer, covered, for 30 to 35 minutes. Do not boil away all of the liquid and do not stir the rice.

3. When a very small amount of liquid remains (about 1 tablespoon), remove the pan from the burner and let it stand, covered, for 3 minutes.

4. While the rice is cooking, heat the oil in a medium-size skillet over medium heat. Add the shallots and cook, stirring occasionally. Add the white part of the green onions and cook for about 1 minute. Add the peppers.

5. Cook for about 5 minutes, stirring frequently. Add the cumin, chili powder, oregano, and cayenne to taste. Cook for about 1 minute, stirring until the spices are well blended.

6. When cooked, set aside until the rice is done. Add the spiced veggies to the rice with the green onion tops, and stir well. Serve.

Maple-Sweetened Collard Greens

SERVINGS: 4 ▌ **SERVING SIZE:** ABOUT ½ CUP GREENS ▌ THIS RECIPE CAN EASILY BE MUL-TIPLIED BY 2, 3, OR 4 ▌ **COOKING TIME:** 15 MINUTES

1 teaspoon grapeseed oil
1 medium-size white onion, diced
1 pound fresh collard greens
2 tablespoons pure maple syrup
1 teaspoon lemon juice
⅛ teaspoon salt
1 teaspoon unsalted butter

NUTRITION FACTS

Serving size about ½ cup greens
Servings 4
Calories 103
Calories from Fat 23
Total Fat 3 g (4%)
Saturated Fat 1 g (4%)
Trans Fat 0 g
Monounsaturated Fat 1 g
Cholesterol 3 mg (1%)
Sodium 101 mg (4%)
Total Carbohydrates 19 g (6%)
Dietary Fiber 5 g (20%)
Sugars 3 g
Protein 3 g
Vitamin A (153%)
Vitamin C (73%)
Calcium (18%)
Iron (2%)

*Parenthetical percentages refer to % Daily Value.

Okay, so you don't think that you like collard greens. Because I was born in the South, I was supposed to like greens, but I didn't. It wasn't until I learned about food that I came to love them.

Collards have to be complemented with other flavors to activate the taste buds. Without a little salt, they are bland and bitter. It is the pure maple syrup that makes this recipe so fantastic. Honey will work fine if you don't have maple syrup, and it will give the finished dish a more flowery flavor. The combination of salty, bitter, and sweet tastes releases the true flavor of the greens.

1. Heat the grapeseed oil in a large skillet over medium heat. Add the onion and cook slowly, for about 20 minutes, until translucent. Stir frequently.

2. While the onion is cooking, wash the collards well and slice into 2-inch squares.

3. Add the collard greens to the pan with the onion and toss. As they begin to wilt, add the maple syrup, lemon juice, salt, and butter. Cook until the collards are hot and wilted, but not to the point that they begin to lose their bright green color.

CONVENIENCE MEALS

Lean Cuisine Szechuan Style Stir Fry with Shrimp or
Lean Cuisine Lemon Pepper Fish

RESTAURANT MEALS

P. F. Chang's Seared Ahi Tuna (sauce on the side) or
P. F. Chang's Cantonese Scallops

DAY 5 | *SET REALISTIC GOALS AND PUT YOUR GOALS IN MOTION*

Everyone has a motivation for picking up a book like this one.

Looking over the most successful titles in the bookstore, it's clear that the number one reason people purchase diet books is to lose weight. There's nothing wrong with that, but for most people this usually means they want to lose a lot of pounds really fast. Those books reinforce the idea by claiming to offer rapid, long-term weight loss.

The problem is even if those diets work, you'll likely regain all the weight you lost, plus some. The landscape is littered with failed diet books and with celebrities who've lost and gained and lost and gained. Studies of these diets have shown that many of those books offer users nothing but a yo-yo pattern of weight loss and weight gain.

This is why I would like you to consider exactly what you are looking to accomplish by changing how you eat.

All successful projects work because they have a goal. This is true whether your goal is to save money, build a house, or eat better. But people don't often explore their motivation for wanting to lose weight. One of the most popular reasons people give for going on a diet is "to be healthier." Second most popular is "the positive effects on appearance and well-being."

As you begin to make changes in your life, it's important for you to figure this out for yourself. What exactly do you want to accomplish? Write down your goals. There has been a lot of research about how people outline change with many different methods. *C* is for change and remembering the five C's will help keep you on track.

1. Be Clear

First and foremost, your plans should be clear. Research shows that when your goals are definite, clear, and have a specific time for completion, you will be more successful.

> I want to feel better because _____.
> My goal weight is ____.
> I will reach my goal on _____.

2. Challenge Yourself Daily

It may seem hokey to put a sticky note on your fridge, in your wallet, or on the bathroom mirror, but these sorts of reminders to yourself have been shown to help you define your motivation and keep your goals at the front of your mind. Research also shows that weighing yourself regularly (weekly at least but daily is better) can help you be more successful at weight loss.

3. Commitment

Commit yourself to long-term success. As I mentioned on Day 4, when I talk to patients about losing weight, they are shocked when I tell them what an ideal weight should be for them. After the shock wears off, they say something like, "Oh, I can do that. I'll lose those fifty pounds this summer. You'll see when I come back in three months."

Man, oh man, do I wish I had a dollar for every time someone said that (and another dollar for those who return in three months and have not lost any weight at all). I have no doubt that this mentality comes from fad diet books and pills that repeatedly claim that people can easily lose that much weight in such a short period. All in all I can't object to the goal of losing 50 pounds, but the idea that they will get there in three months is seriously flawed.

Keep in mind that eating better and being healthier is not about three weeks from now or even three months or three years. *This is about making a significant lifelong change.* Plan for that and you'll be successful, for sure.

Today and every day, you want to recommit to setting your goals in action. If it's eating healthier, take out your calendar and mark off the changes you want to make for each week. Here are some suggestions for each weekly goal as part of the fourth C:

4. Complexity

Research says that you have to create specific goals, but they need to be complex so that they will be challenging enough to keep you engaged. The goal should not be so difficult that it is not feasible for you. Here's some examples of goals with specific steps that can help you be successful:

GOAL: TAKE CONTROL OF MY FOOD (PLANNING)

- Sit down each weekend and plan the twenty-one meals for the coming week.
- Make a shopping list for those meals and buy your great ingredients before the week begins.
- Figure out when you are going to eat out, eat leftovers, or eat frozen meals.

GOAL: EAT HEALTHIER

- Stop drinking soda (including diet soda).
- Throw away (or give away to a local food bank) all processed/boxed foods in your pantry.

- Fill your house with unsalted nuts to snack on.
- Fill your house with fresh fruit to snack on.

GOAL: LOSE WEIGHT

- Start a food diary and write down everything you eat. (See Day 7.)
- Buy a food scale.
- Buy a scale for yourself.
- Write down your target weights for the week on each Monday of your calendar.

GOAL: EXERCISE MORE

- Plan your exercise days. Schedule them just as you would a meeting or other appointment.
- What exercise do you like to do? Whatever it is, plan to do it. Join a gym, get your bicycle out of the garage and get it tuned up, or get a new pair of running or walking shoes.

You get the idea. It's one thing to have a goal—the crucial step is to figure out the steps you will take to get to that goal. Long-term goals are important, but breaking them down into incremental steps can help keep you on track. For instance, if you want to lose 30 pounds, break that down over twelve months at 2½ pounds per month. Or if your goal is to eat more fruit, set a goal of eating an extra piece of fruit each day. Keep it simple and make it work for you.

5. Compensate

This has two meanings. The first is that you need ongoing review of your goals and to compensate for successes you have as well as setbacks. Make adjustments and be flexible. Is your goal so high you can't achieve it? Often this means giving yourself more leeway than you might have started with. Or maybe your goal is too aggressive for long-term success. For instance, if you are losing weight at much more than 2 pounds per week, you might be moving too fast. Liberalizing your diet a bit can help you be more successful for the long haul.

The other meaning for *compensate* is to reward yourself. This must be a *nonfood* reward. After sticking to your plans for four weeks, you should have a tangible reward. Do you want a new pair of shoes? A massage? Plan to compensate yourself as part of your goal. Sometimes these rewards can be made possible by achieving your goals. By taking your lunch each day, the $5 you save adds up to over $1,000 per year, and those can be the funds you use for a great reward.

Clear goals that are challenging and suitably complex are important. Committing to them daily and then compensating by being flexible and also rewarding yourself will result in ongoing success.

DAY 5 | DINNER

LEFTOVER LENTIL CHILI (PAGE 32) AND SALAD WITH TOMATO-CHIVE DRESSING (PAGE 33)

> ### Chef Tim Says . . . Try Spinach Instead of Lettuce
>
> When thinking of greens for a salad, don't limit yourself to lettuces. Spinach makes a great choice because it's so widely available, delicious, and versatile. It works well on sandwiches or burgers, too. Popeye ate spinach because of its high amounts of vitamins A and C, and iron. In addition, spinach has almost three times the fiber of lettuce.
>
> Two main types of spinach are available: flat leaf and curly leaf. For the most part, spinach is spinach, but there are some subtle differences.
>
> Flat leaf: The leaves are flat and slightly plump. They will sometimes have a fine fuzz on them. Flat-leaf spinach is easy to clean (always a plus). The flavor is not quite as sweet as that of curly-leaf spinach.
>
> Curly-leaf spinach is of two kinds. In gardening terms, curly spinach is said to be *savoyed* and can be either semi-savoyed or heavily savoyed. The more curly (savoyed) the spinach is, the harder it is to clean.
>
> In most cooked recipes, frozen spinach works just fine. The time you spend to clean, rinse, and cook fresh spinach is not worth the difference in flavor in a dish such as soup, stuffed shells, or quiche. Place the thawed spinach in a strainer and press with a spoon to squeeze out the excess water.

Day 5 Alternative Dinner Choices

CONVENIENCE MEALS

Amy's Mexican Casserole or
Amy's Tortilla Casserole

RESTAURANT MEALS

Ruby Tuesday Half-Serving Fresh Avocado Quesadilla with a Salad Bar
(take the other half for lunch tomorrow)

DAY 6 | *READJUST YOUR GOALS OVER TIME*

Now that you have considered your goals, I want you understand that they may change over time, depending on where you are in your progress toward long-term success.

The idea of change being a process grows out of work by two researchers, J. O. Prochaska and C. C. DiClemente,[9] and is a model for you to understand "where your head is at." Their idea is that we are always at some point along a continuum of being ready for change. The most basic step is called the Pre-Contemplation Stage. If you are in this stage, you are basically not really thinking that the change is important and your response to the idea of changing your diet or lifestyle would be, "I'm not interested; it doesn't matter."

Here are the seven stages and how they might apply to you and eating healthy (in the past as well as now and the future):

Keep in mind that these stages are fluid. You can move forward and backward along the continuum at different times and it's important to readjust your goals accordingly. You may be in the Action stage with your diet but only the Preparation phase with exercising.

I will discuss creating your own meal plans on Day 18. Remember to sit down once a week to plan the upcoming seven days. That's also a time to consider how you've done, what you have accomplished, and to realign your goals to meet your day-to-day needs.

STAGES

STAGE OF CHANGE	CHARACTERISTICS	DIET IMPACT FOR YOU
PRE-CONTEMPLATION	You are not thinking about change right now.	In this stage, you don't think that changing diet or lifestyle is important. If you bought this book or have read this far, it's likely that you are long past this stage, but someone in your family may not be ready to change and that may be a factor in how you plan to make change for yourself.
CONTEMPLATION	You have thought about change and maybe considered that it is important, but haven't taken steps toward change.	You may now know that diet, healthy lifestyle, and weight loss are important and are considering making a change.
PREPARATION	You are making plans to change and maybe have even set dates, times, and goals for change.	You have likely passed this by now on Day 6 with actually taking action, but it's possible that you have been reading this far and not following the Dr. Gourmet Diet Plan. That's okay. Keep reading and move to the next stage, action.
ACTION	This is where you are taking action to make changes for yourself.	Ideally, you have been in this stage since picking up this book. By opening and reading it, you have taken some action. Only by following the diet and working toward your goals will you be fully in the action stage.
MAINTENANCE	You have an ongoing commitment to your change.	This is the challenging part for many of us. Sometimes it's easy to contemplate, prepare, and take action, but maintaining that action is the key to your long-term success. Return to your goals over and over, to keep yourself on track.
RELAPSE	You are falling back into old habits.	Hey, it happens. We all have setbacks when we are working on changes in our lives. If this happens, return to the preparation stage (keep it short) and then move right back into taking action.

Asian Peanut Chicken with Noodles

SERVINGS: 2 ▌ **SERVING SIZE: 2 OUNCES PASTA WITH CHICKEN AND SAUCE** ▌ **THIS RECIPE CAN EASILY BE MULTIPLIED** ▌ **COOKING TIME: 30 MINUTES**

3 tablespoons smooth peanut butter

¼ cup fresh cilantro leaves

Juice of ½ lime

2 teaspoons low-sodium soy sauce

2 tablespoons low-sodium chicken stock

⅛ teaspoon red pepper flakes

6 ounces boneless, skinless chicken breast, sliced into strips

4 ounces whole wheat spaghetti

½ cup frozen edamame

1 small carrot, shredded

Slivered red onion

2 tablespoons dry-roasted unsalted peanuts

NUTRITION FACTS

Serving size 2 ounces pasta with chicken and sauce
Servings 2
Calories 581
Calories from Fat 190
Total Fat 23 g (35%)
Saturated Fat 4 g (21%)
Trans Fat 0 g
Monounsaturated Fat 9 g
Cholesterol 49 mg (16%)
Sodium 257 mg (11%)
Total Carbohydrates 59 g (20%)
Dietary Fiber 10 g (41%)
Sugars 6 g
Protein 44 g
Vitamin A (49%)
Vitamin C (22%)
Calcium (11%)
Iron (33%)

*Parenthetical percentages refer to % Daily Value.

This recipe makes good leftovers if reheated gently. Leftovers, chilled, work well as a pasta salad.

This peanut chicken recipe is so quick and simple to make. It takes practically no time, is full of flavor, and, compared to ordering takeout, will save you up to 1,000 calories. The recipe calls for whole wheat spaghetti, but the traditional noodles would be buckwheat soba. These are widely available now and delicious. Try them, and when you do, use the package directions for cooking the noodles.

1. Place the peanut butter, cilantro, lime juice, soy sauce, chicken stock, and red pepper flakes in a blender or mini chopper and puree until smooth. Set aside.

2. Preheat the oven to 200°F.

3. Place 3 quarts of water in a large saucepan over high heat. When the water boils, lower the heat to medium until the water is simmering. Add the chicken strips and cook for 5 minutes. Remove the chicken with tongs, leaving the water in the pot, and place the chicken on a heatproof plate in the preheated oven.

4. Increase the heat under the water to high, and when the water returns to a boil, add the pasta. Cook for 8 to 10 minutes, until the pasta is almost al dente. Add the edamame and cook for another minute.

[CONTINUES]

5. Remove ½ cup of the pasta water and reserve. Drain the pasta and edamame, then return to the saucepan. Lower the heat to medium and add the peanut sauce, chicken, and shredded carrot, and slivered onion to taste, then toss well.

6. If the sauce is too thick, add the reserved pasta water, 1 tablespoon at a time, until it reaches the desired consistency. Top with the peanuts and serve.

Dr. Tim Says . . . Be Careful Handling Poultry

It is important to be very careful when handling poultry. Use the freshest chicken or turkey possible. If there is any odd odor at all, don't use it.

Only cut poultry on a plastic cutting board and wash the cutting board, your hands, and your knives in soapy water as soon as you are finished. This reduces the risk of spreading the bacteria to other foods.

Be sure to cook poultry thoroughly. Use a small instant-read thermometer to check for the right temperatures. Whole chicken (or any poultry) should reach 180°F in the thigh or 170°F in the breast. (The recommendation is similar for pieces of cut chicken.)

Free-range chickens have not been proven to be safer. Many of the growers of free-range chickens don't use antibiotics and feed their chickens carefully, but there is no proof yet that this results in a bacteria-free bird. I do think that free-range chickens taste better, however.

Day 6 Alternative Dinner Choices

CONVENIENCE MEALS

Lean Cuisine Chicken in Peanut Sauce or
Kashi Sweet and Sour Chicken

RESTAURANT MEALS

Applebee's Tortilla Chicken Melt

DAY 7 | *KEEP A DIET AND EXERCISE DIARY*

Tracking what you eat has long been the foundation of successful weight-loss programs because it helps you learn exactly how many calories you are eating. It also helps you identify where you can improve the quality of the calories that you are consuming. You'll also see in black and white just what's in your meals and gain a better understanding of what a normal portion size is.

I have seen firsthand how well keeping a food diary can work for patients, and there's good research showing that those who are both truthful and thorough have long term success at both losing weight and keeping it off. One study[10] compared different tools people used to lose weight and found that using a food diary was shown to be more powerful than exercise is for long-term successful weight loss! Those in the study who faithfully kept a food diary lost twice as much weight as those who didn't.

Keeping a food diary is free, easy, and takes only a few minutes a day. You'll quickly find that keeping track of what you eat is one of the most important tools you have.

You're not limited to using only pen and paper. Most of us are used to computers, iPhones, mobile phones, and other handheld devices. Dozens of Web sites (including DrGourmet.com) now offer online food diaries or applications you can install on your phone or other handheld device. In fact, one study[11] showed that using a Web site to track calories can really work well. In other research, participants did well using only a photographic food diary. It appears that simply taking a picture of what you eat before you eat it can help you lose weight.[12]

When I talk with my patients about keeping a food diary, I encourage them to keep track of their exercise and their weight as well. Those who record their weight regularly tend to stay on track,[13] and I think that knowing how much you are exercising encourages you to work harder and compete with yourself to do a little more each week. We also know that keeping track of your weight on a regular basis helps you to lose the weight in the first place, in addition to keeping it off.[14]

In my practice, those patients who have kept track of their intake and their weight have always done the best at losing weight and keeping it off. Those who plan ahead do even better. If you already know what you are going to eat in the coming week, your food diary is essentially already filled out. All you need to do is follow it and add any changes you might make during the week.

Barbecue Chicken Pizza

SERVINGS: 1 ▮ **SERVING SIZE:** 1 INDIVIDUAL PIZZA ▮ THIS RECIPE CAN EASILY BE MULTI-PLIED ▮ **PREP TIME:** 30 MINUTES ▮ **TOTAL TIME:** 120 MINUTES

Spray olive oil
1 medium-size onion, sliced
3 ounces boneless, skinless chicken breast
¼ cup barbecue sauce (recipe follows)
¼ whole wheat pizza dough recipe (recipe follows), or 1 whole wheat pita round
4 ounces cherry or grape tomatoes, cut into quarters
1 ounce reduced-fat Monterey Jack cheese, shredded

NUTRITION FACTS

Serving size 1 pizza
Servings 1
Calories 584
Calories from Fat 78
Total Fat 9 g (14%)
Saturated Fat 5 g (23%)
Trans Fat 0 g
Monounsaturated Fat 2 g
Cholesterol 67 mg (22%)
Sodium 562 mg (23%)
Total Carbohydrates 90 g (30%)
Dietary Fiber 11 g (46%)
Sugars 23 g
Protein 40 g
Vitamin A (8%)
Vitamin C (35%)
Calcium (30%)
Iron (30%)

*Parenthetical percentages refer to % Daily Value.

Most people think of pizza as not being very healthy. This can be true in places like fast-food pizza chains, where pizzas are made with poor-quality ingredients such as white flour; sauces that are high in fat, calories, and salt; as well as highly processed meats and cheeses.

But you can make great, delicious, healthy pizza so easily. Use whole wheat dough, lower-calorie sauces with less sodium, fresh veggies and meats, and great-quality cheeses. If you don't have time to make pizza dough, in a pinch, use a whole wheat pita round instead.

1. Preheat the oven to 325°F. Place a pizza stone in the oven and place a medium-size ovenproof skillet on top of the pizza stone.

2. Place a large nonstick skillet over medium-high heat and spray lightly with olive oil. Add the onion and cook until well browned. Set aside.

3. When the oven is preheated, place the chicken breast in the skillet that has preheated in the oven and set it back in the oven on top of the pizza stone. Roast on each side for 8 to 10 minutes, then remove the skillet from the oven. Increase the heat in the oven to 500°F.

4. Place the chicken breast on a cutting board and cut into small strips. Place the chicken strips in a bowl and add the barbecue sauce. Toss well to coat the chicken with the sauce.

[CONTINUES]

5. While the chicken is roasting, roll out the pizza dough. Top the dough with the onion and then the tomatoes. Spread the barbecued chicken over the top and place the pizza directly on the pizza stone in the oven.

6. Cook for 5 to 7 minutes and turn the pizza around in case there are any hot spots in the oven. Before turning, sprinkle the shredded cheese over the top.

7. Cook for another 5 to 7 minutes, until the cheese is melted and the crust is golden brown. Serve.

Chef Tim Says . . . Get a Pizza Stone

If you are going to make pizza regularly (and you should—it can be really healthy), then buy a pizza stone. These come in both round and rectangular shapes and are made with everything from ceramic to clay to different mixtures of cement. The cement ones seem to be more durable, as I have broken more than a few ceramic pizza stones.

Place the stone in a cold oven and set the temperature to 500°F. It will take about 20 minutes to heat the oven and stone together. I generally place my shaped pizza dough directly on the stone and then add the toppings. You can also use a peel (the large paddle you see in pizza restaurants) and assemble the pizza on the peel prior to sliding it onto the stone.

By using a pizza stone, the heat will be transferred evenly to your pizza, crisping the crust. Over time, the stone will darken. When you are done cooking your pizza, simply shut off the oven and let the stone cool. I don't use water on mine but simply brush it off or use a spatula to scrape off anything that has stuck to the stone.

Whole Wheat Pizza Dough

SERVINGS: ENOUGH DOUGH FOR 4 INDIVIDUAL PIZZAS ▌ **SERVING SIZE:** 1 INDIVIDUAL PIZZA ▌ THIS RECIPE IS EASILY DOUBLED OR HALVED ▌ **COOKING TIME:** 90 MINUTES

1 teaspoon dry active yeast
4 teaspoons honey
2 cups whole wheat flour
(does not need to be sifted)
½ cup all-purpose flour
(does not need to be sifted)
½ teaspoon salt

NUTRITION FACTS

Serving size 1 pizza
Servings 4
Calories 284
Calories from Fat 9
Total Fat 1 g (5%)
Saturated Fat 0 g (0%)
Trans Fat 0 g
Monounsaturated Fat 0 g
Cholesterol 0 mg (0%)
Sodium 295 mg (12%)
Total Carbohydrates 61 g (20%)
Dietary Fiber 8 g (32%)
Sugars 6 g
Protein 10 g
Vitamin A (0%)
Vitamin C (0%)
Calcium (2%)
Iron (18%)

*Parenthetical percentages refer to % Daily Value.

Using whole wheat pizza dough for pizza recipes is a great way to get extra fiber. The dough has more body than regular pizza dough and a mellow, sweet flavor. And it adds 6 grams of fiber to your diet!

This dough will keep for about 36 hours in the refrigerator if wrapped tightly in plastic wrap, although it will not be as good as fresh.

1. Heat 1 cup of water in the microwave until warm to touch—110°F to 115°F. (I prefer to use a thermometer for this because if the water is too hot, you will kill the yeast.)

2. Place the yeast and honey in a large mixing bowl and pour the heated water over the mixture, stirring until well blended. Let the mixture stand for 5 to 7 minutes, until foamy.

3. Add the whole wheat flour, all-purpose flour, and salt and stir with a fork until a coarse dough forms. Continue to mix by hand until a dough ball forms and all the flour is well blended.

4. Cover the bowl and place it in a sink that has about 4 inches of hot water in the bottom. The heat from the warm water will help the dough rise. The dough will double in size in 30 to 40 minutes. Punch it a few times with your fingers and let it rise another 30 minutes.

5. Remove the dough from the bowl and cut the ball into four equal pieces. Cover the dough that you are not going to use immediately in plastic wrap and chill.

up-to-date research shows that *consuming fewer calories is the only way to lose weight*. I do also want you to learn to identify better nutritional-quality calories, because being healthy is partly about weight loss and partly about the types of food you eat. Understanding the truth about fats, carbohydrates, and other macronutrients is the key to eating the best-quality calories. You might think that these are the enemy—but fat *is* good for you and so are carbohydrates, and I'll show you how to choose the right ones.

This week's menu includes familiar dishes such as cashew chicken and Philly cheese steak sandwiches, but I also want you to expand your horizons a bit, so I've included recipes with such ingredients as eggplant and risotto as well as techniques that are quick and easy and that produce delicious results, such as cooking fish wrapped in foil.

This week, you'll:

▌ Understand calories and important macronutrients:

Saturated fats	Unhealthy trans fats
Healthy fats	Carbohydrates

▌ Learn about soluble and insoluble fiber
▌ Expand your techniques, including:

Cooking in foil	Cooking beef
Creative use of leftovers	Making risotto

Chef Tim Says . . . Rest Your Meat After Cooking

When cooking meats, it is important to remove them from the heat a little early. After removing meat from the oven or grill, the internal temperature of the meat continues to rise (some people call this "carryover cooking"). Without the continued high temperature of the oven, the external temperature of the meat decreases, however, and the result is redistribution of the juices in the meat, making it both easier to carve as well as more succulent.

Flank steak should be allowed to "rest" for 3 to 5 minutes, but a larger cut needs to rest for at least 7 to 10 minutes. If you are cooking with an instant-read thermometer, figure that the internal temperature in a smaller piece of meat will increase by about 15°F and a larger piece by about 10°F while it rests. For example, after cooking a pork tenderloin to 135°F in the oven, the temperature will rise to 145° to 150°F as it rests.

A personalized shopping list for Week 2 can be found at DrGourmet .com/shoppinglist.

WEEK 2 MENU

RECIPE	CONVENIENCE FOOD ALTERNATIVE	RESTAURANT MEAL ALTERNATIVE
DAY 8		
Fettuccine with Roasted Eggplant and Broccoli	Lean Cuisine Penne Pasta with Tomato Basil Sauce or Weight Watchers Smart Ones Lasagna Florentine	Ruby Tuesday Asian Dumplings with Salad Bar
DAY 9		
Garlic-Lime Flank Steak, Mashed Yams, and Herbed Zucchini	Weight Watchers Spaghetti with Meat Sauce (Spaghetti Bolognese)	Ruby Tuesday Petite Sirloin with a Side Salad
DAY 10		
Cashew Chicken	Lean Cuisine Chicken in Peanut Sauce	Red Lobster Shrimp Cocktail Appetizer with a Side Salad and Baked Potato
DAY 11		
Whitefish in Foil with Vegetables and Tomato Sauce and Caesar Salad	Lean Cuisine Lemon Pepper Fish or Lean Cuisine Szechuan Style Stir Fry with Shrimp	Ruby Tuesday Asian Glazed Salmon
DAY 12		
Philly Cheese Steak and Waldorf Salad	Lean Cuisine Chicken, Spinach, and Mushroom Panini or Lean Cuisine Southwest-Style Chicken Panini	Panera Bread Half-Serving Chicken Tomesto on French Bread with a Large Fresh Fruit Cup
DAY 13		
Salmon-Squash Risotto	Lean Cuisine Szechuan Style Stir Fry with Shrimp	Panera Boston Clam Chowder with a Large Fresh Fruit Cup
DAY 14		
Leftover Salmon-Squash Risotto	Lean Cuisine Salmon with Basil	Red Lobster Grilled Fish

So far we've gone over getting your day structured for eating breakfast and lunch as well as what makes sense for dinner. All of this takes some planning on your part, and I believe that this is the most important part of being healthy. The better you plan, the more likely it is that you will stick to eating healthy.

People will plan almost every aspect of their lives. They know when they have to be at work, what meetings they will go to, times for the kid's soccer game, when they are going to mow the lawn, and on and on. Any successful project requires a plan. You wouldn't think of building a house without architectural drawings and a construction plan. But people just don't take the time to put their meals into their plans, so they end up stopping off at Burger King or standing in front of the fridge at 6:00 PM, thinking, "What are we gonna have for dinner?"

This book provides you with six weeks of meal plans, but you will need to figure out how to fit them into your life. If you know that you will be running late on Tuesday, that's a good day to eat out or have a convenience meal. The single most important thing you can do for eating healthy and losing weight is to know what you are going to eat and when—*in advance.*

This is something that you will need to do every week. Pick a day, sit down, and sketch out what you are going to have for the upcoming twenty-one meals. It's also a good idea to plan for your snacks. If you are a sweet snacker, put fresh or dried fruit on your shopping list. If you are a salty/savory snacker, try nuts or those 100-calorie packs of popcorn.

This means you'll have what you need on hand for breakfast and lunch. And remember, it takes just a minute or two to make a sandwich before leaving for work, plus you'll save a huge number of calories each week. And think of all the money you'll save—as much as $30 per week and about $1,500 per year.

You can save even more by planning your dinners. Your meal plan should include fish (unless you are allergic to it) three days per week if possible. Eating fish two or more days per week cuts your risk of heart disease by a fairly large amount. Add a meal based on red meat one day per week, and alternate between poultry or vegetarian meals on the other two or three days.

Your dinner menu plan over the first fourteen days should then look much like this:

2 red meat   3 poultry   3 meatless   6 fish

You don't have to create a complete meal from scratch every night. For vegetarian night, this is as easy as making some whole wheat pasta and putting bottled spaghetti sauce and grated Parmesan on it. On the weekends, making soup or chili will give you two or three meals from leftovers later on in the week.

One of the most important parts of your menu planning should be your rewards. *They should not be food rewards!* So often people will make progress, eat better, lose weight, and then turn to food for their reward. Don't. Pick something that you love and use that as your reward. Shoes, movies, vacations, a trip to the spa, or new golf clubs. Plan for something to reward yourself with and you'll stay on track.

Planning your week's meals is the most important step you can take toward being and eating healthier.

Chef Tim Says . . . How to Cook Pasta

Most pastas are named for their shape. For instance, *conchiglie* is the Italian word for "shells." Others include *vermicelli* (small worms), *orzo* (barley), *farfalle* (butterflies), *eliche* (spirals), *cappelletti* (little hats), and so on.

Cooking pasta is really easy, but there are a few techniques that will make your dish better. First and foremost, bring the water to a full boil before adding the pasta and keep the water boiling. When you add the pasta, the water will cool a bit. Cover the pot and when the water is back to a rolling boil, you can uncover it partially by moving the lid just a little to one side. Second, you should check the pasta for doneness by tasting it and stop cooking when it is still a little bit chewy. I *never* rinse pasta. It strips away the lovely carbohydrates that are going to help your sauce be creamier. If for some reason you were going to cook the pasta in advance, you could add ½ teaspoon of oil to the drained pasta and toss to keep it from sticking together.

Notice that this recipe uses some of the pasta water. All great restaurants use this technique and it adds a bit of pasta flavor and a little thickening for your sauce.

Fettuccine with Roasted Eggplant and Broccoli

SERVINGS: 2 ▮ **SERVING SIZE:** 2 OUNCES PASTA WITH VEGGIES ▮ THIS RECIPE CAN EAS-
ILY BE MULTIPLIED ▮ **COOKING TIME:** 60 MINUTES

2 (8-ounce) eggplants
8 ounces broccoli
Spray olive oil
4 ounces whole wheat
    fettuccine
1 tablespoon olive oil
1 clove garlic, minced
1 tablespoon pine nuts
1 teaspoon lemon zest
2 tablespoons balsamic
    vinegar
¼ teaspoon salt
Freshly ground black
    pepper
2 tablespoons flat-leaf
    parsley leaves
1 ounce aged Gruyère
    cheese (Asiago or other
    hard cheese will do)

NUTRITION FACTS

Serving size 2 ounces pasta
    with veggies
Servings 2
Calories 472
Calories from Fat 155
Total Fat 18 g (28%)
Saturated Fat 4 g (21%)
Trans Fat 0 g
Monounsaturated Fat 8 g
Cholesterol 16 mg (5%)
Sodium 388 mg (16%)
Total Carbohydrates 67 g (22%)
Dietary Fiber 11 g (45%)
Sugars 10 g
Protein 19 g
Vitamin A (25%)
Vitamin C (189%)
Calcium (25%)
Iron (23%)

*Parenthetical percentages
refer to % Daily Value.

Meatless meals are a great way to be healthier and to lose weight. One of my favorite ingredients for vegetarian dishes is eggplant. Its rich, savory flavor is perfect and it's so filling along with a good-quality cheese. This is a recipe that is both delicious and satisfying.

1. Cut the eggplants lengthwise and then cut each piece lengthwise again. Cut the quartered eggplant across so that you have cubes about 1 inch across. Cut the broccoli so that each floret has a long, tapered stem.

2. Preheat the oven to 325°F and place a large ovenproof sauté pan or grill pan inside.

3. Fit a medium-size saucepan with a steamer basket and place 1 cup of water in the bottom of the pot. Place the eggplant in the steamer and then top with the broccoli florets. Place the pot over high heat and steam the vegetables for 7 minutes.

4. Remove the broccoli and eggplant and set the eggplant on a plate to cool. Transfer the broccoli to the large, preheated skillet and spray lightly with olive oil. Place the pan in the oven and roast the broccoli for 7 to 10 minutes.

5. Remove the broccoli and again spray lightly with olive oil. Place the eggplant in the skillet, return the pan to the oven, and roast for about 40 minutes. The key to this recipe is cooking the eggplant long enough that the inside is creamy and the skin is slightly browned with a roasted flavor. Just as the eggplant seems to be getting soft is the time to start the pasta water.

6. After the eggplant has been cooking for about 30 minutes, place 3 quarts of water in a medium-size stockpot over high heat. When the water is boiling, add the fettuccine. Cook at a slow boil, stirring occasionally.

7. After about 35 minutes, heat the tablespoon of olive oil in a large skillet over medium heat. Add the garlic, pine nuts, and lemon zest. Cook for about 3 minutes, stirring frequently.

8. Using tongs, remove the cooked fettuccine from the boiling water and add it to the pan. Add the vinegar and salt and pepper to taste. Add ⅓ cup of the water that the pasta boiled in and then add the cooked broccoli and eggplant. Toss the fettuccine and vegetables together for about 2 minutes and add the parsley leaves.

9. Serve topped with ½ ounce of the Gruyère grated over each serving.

Dr. Tim Says . . . Eat Eggplant, It's Great for You!

Eggplant belongs to the nightshade family, along with tomatoes and potatoes. The large, dark purple, pear-shaped eggplant is the most common kind. There are virtually no calories in eggplant (about 20 calories in a cup of raw fruit). It has very little fat but has tons of fiber (2 grams per cup).

The larger the eggplant, the milder the flavor and the tougher the skin. I generally look for fruit no more than about 1 pound (about 8 inches long and 4 inches in diameter).

The much smaller version of the dark purple eggplant is often called Italian or baby eggplant. These are more flavorful and the flesh is somewhat more tender.

The straight, thin eggplant known as Japanese or Asian eggplant has a thin delicate skin, like Italian eggplant, but the flesh is sweeter. The color ranges from dark purple to a striped purple as well as light amethyst. Because of the sweet flavor and delicate texture, this is the type that I recommend using for any dishes where I may want whole slices or chunks (such as ratatouille).

White-skinned eggplant is now widely available and it is actually this variety that gave eggplant its common name. Also delicate in flavor, it is especially beautiful when grilled.

Day 8 Alternative Dinner Choices

CONVENIENCE MEALS

Lean Cuisine Penne Pasta with Tomato Basil Sauce or
　　Weight Watchers Smart Ones Lasagna Florentine

RESTAURANT MEALS

Ruby Tuesday Asian Dumplings with Salad Bar

"Just what the heck is a calorie and what do I do with it?!" I hear this a lot from my patients, and knowing the answer is the basis for success in eating well and losing weight.

The calorie is a unit of measure of energy that we use for food. Think of calories as you might the miles per gallon (mpg) fuel economy of your car. If your car gets 20 mpg and the tank holds 10 gallons, you can travel 200 miles before you'll run out of gas. The difference is that, unlike gasoline, different ingredients give you a different mpg. Fats might, for instance, take you farther than carbohydrates in the same way that a premium gasoline might let you drive farther than would a tank full of regular gas. One challenge for us is that our gas tank holds a limited amount of fuel. Our body, however, has an almost unlimited ability to store the excess calories that we consume. Think of this as if your car could keep sprouting more gas tanks as you kept pumping in gasoline.

I will return to the idea of *quality* calories over and over. Although it is important for you to control the number of calories you consume, to lose weight, the types of calories you consume can help you eat fewer calories but actually eat more food. For instance, a tiny breakfast bar that contains 240 calories is only four or five bites. A scrambled egg sandwich is nearly the same number of bites at about 280 calories. The sandwich has great quality carbohydrates from the whole wheat bread, along with protein and fats that will help you remain satisfied through the morning. The breakfast bar, on the other hand, is mostly sugar with some fiber and it contains very little protein to keep you satisfied.

The other end of the spectrum is the sausage biscuit for breakfast. Lower-quality, highly processed white flour is combined with lard or shortening for the biscuit, and it's served with sausage that's high in saturated fat and salt. The scrambled egg sandwich is just as good, if not better tasting, but the sausage biscuit is 480 calories and has only 2 grams of fiber (more about fiber on Day 14). The biscuit has twice as many calories for the same volume of food, and because it is high in fat and salt and low in fiber, the biscuit won't sustain you as well as the scrambled egg sandwich will, so it's likely that you'll be hungry sooner (maybe for another sausage biscuit).

Those additional calories are stored—for the most part as fat cells. By eating better-quality food, you can be satisfied for longer and thus eat fewer calories per day, while actually getting to eat more food by volume.

For the first week of this plan, everyone eats the same number of calories: about 1,200 per day. The recipes and meal plans are designed to be very satisfying, and by using the best ingredient choices I can limit the calories but not limit the flavor. The 1,200-calorie meal plan in the first week does help you get your weight loss jump-started, but it is also designed to show you that you can have great food *and* limit your caloric intake. Not everyone needs the same amount of calories, however. A five-foot-four-inch woman needs far less fuel (calories) than does a six-foot-two-inch male. (The difference between a compact car and a big pickup truck. The truck just gets fewer miles per gallon.) Keep in mind that you have to have enough fuel so that you don't "run out of gas," but at the same time you don't want to "overfill the tank" and gain weight. These six weeks of meal plans and the instructions that go with them are designed to help you get it just right for you. So what should you eat and how will you figure portion sizes for yourself as you go forward in this plan? It's pretty simple, really.

Go to the BMI tables we looked at on Day 4 and review your ideal body weight. Multiply that ideal body weight by 11. Let's say that your ideal body weight is 145 pounds. You'll need about 1,600 calories each day for keeping things going (145 × 11 = 1,595). That's your baseline caloric needs (sometimes called your *basal metabolic rate*) or what you need each day to function.

For most people, it doesn't take many extra calories each day to add on pounds (or lose them). Of all the nutrition concepts that I'll discuss, when it comes to losing weight and maintaining your weight loss, the most important thing for you to focus on is this one: calories. It's more important than fats, more important than protein, more important than carbs.

To lose about ½ pound each week, you'll need to eat 250 calories less than your baseline caloric needs every day. So if you should weigh 145 pounds, you'll need to eat about 1,350 calories per day (1595 − 250 =

SERVING SIZES

CALORIES PER DAY	BREAKFAST (about 250 calories per serving)	LUNCH (about 250 calories per serving)	DINNER (about 500 calories per serving)
1,000	1 serving	1 serving	1 serving
1,200	1 serving	2 servings	1 serving
1,500	2 servings	2 servings	1 serving
1,800	2 servings	2 servings	1½ servings
2,000	2 servings	2 servings	2 servings

1,350) to lose weight. (You can do this by eating 1,595 calories per day and burning those 250 calories by exercising—and you should—as I mentioned in the introduction.)

Translating those calories to meals can be the challenging part of this. The first week, I gave you the outline of what a "serving" might be for breakfast. Generally speaking, if you target about 250 calories for a "serving" at breakfast and lunch and 500 calories at dinner, you'll be able to keep track of your calories more easily. Here's a table to show you how many servings of a typical breakfast, lunch, or dinner meal will add up to the different daily caloric intakes.

The breakfast and lunch servings were explained on Days 1 and 2. For now, follow the recipes to begin understanding what a dinner serving is. In the case of today's dinner, a single serving comes to 2 ounces of pasta with the veggies, nuts, and cheese. The recipes have been created to help you understand the right serving sizes or portions that you should eat at dinner, but I will go into this in much more detail on Day 20.

Note that there is a row for 1,000 calories. Very few people should be on such a low-calorie diet and I only recommend this to certain patients. The body's metabolism slows at that level of caloric intake and it can actually be more difficult to lose weight. Before starting a 1,000-calorie-per-day diet, check with your doctor.

DAY 9 | DINNER

GARLIC-LIME FLANK STEAK, MASHED YAMS, AND HERBED ZUCCHINI

Garlic-Lime Flank Steak

SERVINGS: 3 ▌ **SERVING SIZE:** 4 OUNCES STEAK ▌ THIS RECIPE CAN EASILY BE HALVED
OR MULTIPLIED ▌ **COOKING TIME:** 60 MINUTES

2 tablespoons minced
   shallot
2 cloves garlic, minced
1 tablespoon fresh rosemary
1 tablespoon extra-virgin
   olive oil
1 tablespoon freshly
   squeezed lime juice
½ teaspoon salt
¾ pound flank steak
Spray olive oil

NUTRITION FACTS

Serving size 4 ounces
Servings 3
Calories 218
Calories from Fat 105
Total Fat 12 g (18%)
Saturated Fat 4 g (18%)
Trans Fat 0 g
Monounsaturated Fat 6 g
Cholesterol 48 mg (16%)
Sodium 454 mg (19%)
Total Carbohydrates 2 g (1%)
Dietary Fiber 0 g (0%)
Sugars 0 g
Protein 23 g
Vitamin A (2%)
Vitamin C (4%)
Calcium (4%)
Iron (11%)

*Parenthetical percentages
refer to % Daily Value.

This is a perfect recipe to experiment with. Use a different herb or acid in the marinade each time you make it for a much different flavor. Try dried tarragon and orange juice, or lemon juice and fresh thyme. The combinations are endless. You might not think that beef is good for you, but the problem is not red meat but highly processed red meat. Good-quality, lean flank steak is not the red meat you need to avoid. We now know it is bologna and hot dogs that cause health problems. On Day 30, I will show you evidence that eating beef is okay and just how much and how often you should eat it.

Leftover steak keeps for two to three days and is great on sandwiches. Save one dinner serving for tomorrow's Philly Cheese Steak Sandwich.

1. Combine the shallot, garlic, rosemary, olive oil, lime juice, salt, and flank steak in a zippered plastic bag. Close the bag and toss to coat the steak well. Marinate for at least 4 hours in the refrigerator (overnight is best).

2. When you are ready to cook the steak, preheat the oven to broil or start the barbecue grill on medium-high heat.

3. Lightly spray a broiler or grill pan with oil. Put the flank steak on the pan and place it under the broiler (or place the steak on the grill). Discard the marinade. Cook for 8 to 9 minutes on each side for medium-rare.

4. Transfer to a cutting board and allow the meat to rest for 5 to 10 minutes prior to slicing. Carve the meat as thinly as possible and serve.

Mashed Yams

SERVINGS: 4 ▌ **SERVING SIZE:** ABOUT 1 CUP ▌ THIS RECIPE CAN EASILY BE DOUBLED OR TRIPLED ▌ **COOKING TIME:** 25 MINUTES

1 pound yams, peeled and cubed
1 teaspoon extra-virgin olive oil
1 large shallot, minced
¼ teaspoon dried rosemary
¼ teaspoon salt
Freshly ground black pepper
2 tablespoons light spread, such as Take Control or Promise
¼ cup nonfat buttermilk
2 tablespoons 2% milk

NUTRITION FACTS

Serving size 1 cup
Servings 4
Calories 188
Calories from Fat 37
Total Fat 4 g (6%)
Saturated Fat 1 g (5%)
Trans Fat 0 g
Monounsaturated Fat 2 g
Cholesterol 1 mg (<1%)
Sodium 215 mg (9%)
Total Carbohydrates 35 g (12%)
Dietary Fiber 5 g (19%)
Sugars 2 g
Protein 3 g
Vitamin A (14%)
Vitamin C (35%)
Calcium (6%)
Iron (4%)
Vitamin K 6 mcg
Potassium 1,021 mg
Magnesium 31 mg

*Parenthetical percentages refer to % Daily Value.

Mashed yams make a delicious alternative to potatoes. They have much the same texture but so much more character and more fiber. Dishes like this will make your main course really special.

This recipe makes good leftovers and will keep well in the refrigerator for about 48 hours. Reheat gently.

1. Place 1 quart of water in a large stockpot fitted with a steamer basket over high heat.

2. Add the cubed yams to the steamer basket and steam until they break slightly with a fork.

3. While the yams are cooking, place the olive oil in a small skillet over medium heat. Add the shallots and rosemary and cook gently until the shallots are softened.

4. Place the cooked yams together with the shallot and rosemary mixture in a bowl. Add the salt, pepper to taste, spread, and buttermilk, and mash with a fork until smooth. Add the 2% milk slowly as the yams are mashed smooth.

> **Dr. Tim Says . . .**
> Choosing yams instead of potatoes in your favorite recipe brings a whole new level of healthy to your table. Yams have 50 percent more fiber than potatoes do, so they will stay with you longer. They are also a rich source of vitamins C and B$_6$, and potassium.

Herbed Zucchini

SERVINGS: 4 ▍ **SERVING SIZE:** ABOUT ⅔ CUP ▍ THIS RECIPE CAN EASILY BE DOUBLED, USING A LARGE SKILLET ▍ **COOKING TIME:** 20 MINUTES

1 tablespoon olive oil
1 pound zucchini, cut into ¼-inch dice
2 tablespoons fresh herbs of your choice, minced
¼ teaspoon salt
Freshly ground black pepper

NUTRITION FACTS

Serving size about ⅔ cup
Servings 4
Calories 51
Calories from Fat 32
Total Fat 4 g (6%)
Saturated Fat 1 g (3%)
Trans Fat 0 g
Monounsaturated Fat 3 g
Cholesterol 0 mg (0%)
Sodium 88 mg (4%)
Total Carbohydrates 5 g (2%)
Dietary Fiber 2 g (7%)
Sugars 2 g
Protein 2 g
Vitamin A (6%)
Vitamin C (33%)
Calcium (4%)
Iron (8%)

*Parenthetical percentages refer to % Daily Value.

The choice of herbs here is not important, as long as you use fresh herbs. Use what you have in the garden or the fridge. Equal amounts of basil, chive, sage, rosemary, and oregano will do, but you could just as easily choose thyme, sage, marjoram, and tarragon. This recipe will work with dried herbs but the flavor just isn't quite as good.

1. Place the olive oil in a large nonstick skillet over medium-high heat. When the oil is hot, add the zucchini. Let the zucchini cook without stirring for about 3 minutes. If it appears to be cooking too fast, lower the heat to medium.

2. Toss the zucchini well and cook for 7 to 10 more minutes. As the cubes begin to brown, add the herbs, salt, and pepper to taste, and continue to toss.

3. Do not overcook the zucchini. As soon as the outside is lightly browned and it is slightly soft, serve.

> **Dr. Tim Says . . .**
> Zucchini are delicious, versatile, and great for you. A large zucchini has almost a full day's requirement of vitamin C, is full of fiber, and has only about 50 calories.

CONVENIENCE MEALS

Weight Watchers Spaghetti with Meat Sauce (Spaghetti Bolognese)

RESTAURANT MEALS

Ruby Tuesday Petite Sirloin with a Side Salad

DAY 10 | EAT FEWER CALORIES, LOSE WEIGHT!

There has been so much debate about what is the best way to lose weight, it's no wonder people don't know what to eat. First we were told to eat a low-carb diet, then that lowering our fat intake would work. Then there were diets with all different ratios: high protein/low fat, low carb/high fat, super low fat/high carb.

I've seen a lot of studies on all types of diets, and the results have been a bit confusing. The research often doesn't last long enough (six months or less), or doesn't include a good mix of men and women. Sometimes it includes far too few people to draw any reliable conclusions.

Researchers recently created a study with an eye to overcoming those common problems so they could try to answer the question of what combination of protein, fat, and carbohydrates is best for sustained weight loss.[1] They recruited 645 overweight men and women for a two-year weight-loss program. Each person was randomly assigned to one of four diets:

FOUR DIETS	
Low fat with average protein:	20% fat, 15% protein, 65% carbohydrates
Low fat with high protein:	20% fat, 25% protein, 55% carbohydrates
High fat with average-protein:	40% fat, 15% protein, 45% carbohydrates
High fat with high protein:	40% fat, 25% protein, 35% carbohydrates

The four plans were all healthy diets, in that they were low in saturated fat, high in fiber, and low in cholesterol. The participants were taught to choose healthier carbohydrates regardless of the amount of carbs they were assigned to eat.

Each person did some form of moderate exercise for about 90 minutes per week and attended regular support sessions. The participants also received customized meal plans in two-week blocks that aimed to cut their daily calories by 750 calories (that's a lot). They also tracked their calories with an online food and exercise journal.

During the first six months, all of the participants lost about the same amount of weight, no matter which diet they were on, and after the first year, everyone regained about the same amount of weight. After two years, one-third of the study subjects—from all four of the different diets—had lost at least 5 percent of their body weight—and kept it off throughout the study.

Finally! This is evidence that when it comes to weight loss, it doesn't really matter what ratio of fat, protein, or carbohydrates you eat—as long as you eat fewer calories.

Does the ratio matter? It appears that it does. On the one hand, we now know that these ratios of the macronutrients, fat, carbohydrate, and protein don't matter much, when it comes to initial weight loss. It does appear to matter for long-term weight loss and the makeup of your diet does have an effect on other risk factors, such as high blood pressure and heart disease. The issue is twofold: First, you need to find the right number of calories that works for you and your successful weight loss. Second, and more important, is to find a way to eat that allows you to sustain that weight loss for a long, long time. The recipes you are cooking and eating and the information you will continue to read will help you understand the best balance for sustained weight loss and your health.

In short, the type of diet you follow does matter for your overall health, but one of the most important things for you to remember is that by eating fewer calories, you'll be able to lose weight and keep it off.

Cashew Chicken

SERVINGS: 4 ▌ **SERVING SIZE:** ABOUT 1½ CUPS OVER RICE ▌ THIS RECIPE CAN EASILY BE MULTIPLIED ▌ **COOKING TIME:** 30 MINUTES ▌ THIS KEEPS WELL FOR ABOUT 48 HOURS IN THE FRIDGE. REHEAT GENTLY.

1 cup frozen shelled edamame (soybeans)
1 cup uncooked brown rice
2 teaspoons dark sesame oil
1 medium-size white onion, diced
1 clove garlic, minced
1 pound boneless, skinless chicken breast, cut into strips
½ cup raw cashews
1 tablespoon peeled and minced fresh ginger
½ cup low-sodium chicken stock
2 tablespoons low-sodium soy sauce
1 tablespoon pure maple syrup

NUTRITION FACTS

Serving size 1½ cups
Servings 4
Calories 529
Calories from Fat 145
Total Fat 17 g (26%)
Saturated Fat 3 g (16%)
Trans Fat 0 g
Monounsaturated Fat 7 g
Cholesterol 65 mg (22%)
Sodium 391 mg (16%)
Total Carbohydrates 55 g (18%)
Dietary Fiber 6 g (22%)
Sugars 8 g
Protein 41 g
Vitamin A (1%)
Vitamin C (9%)
Calcium (9%)
Iron (26%)

*Parenthetical percentages refer to % Daily Value.

A recipe like this can easily have as much as 80 grams of fat per serving in an Asian restaurant! At the same time, the Chinese takeout will come with white rice and a ton of added sodium. By comparison, this one has half the calories, one-fourth the fat and sodium, and three times as much fiber. This is a great example of quality calories—healthy ingredient choices such as brown rice, rich and flavorful sesame oil, and cashews come together in a quick and easy recipe that you know and love (and you'll love it even more when you think about all the calories you save).

1. Remove the edamame from the freezer, place in a colander, and rinse with cool water. Set aside.

2. In a medium-size saucepan, heat 2 cups of water to a boil, then stir in the brown rice. Lower the heat to medium-low and simmer, partially covered, for 25 to 30 minutes. Do not boil away all of the liquid and do not stir the rice.

3. When a very small amount of liquid remains, remove the pan from the burner and let it stand, covered.

4. While the rice is cooking, place 1 teaspoon of the dark sesame oil in a large nonstick skillet over medium heat. Add the diced onion and cook gently, stirring occasionally. Do not allow the onion to brown; it should cook until soft and translucent. This will take at least 10 minutes. Transfer the onion to a bowl and set aside.

5. Add the other teaspoon of dark sesame oil to the pan with the minced garlic. Cook gently over medium heat for about 5 minutes, until the garlic is soft. Do not let the garlic brown.

6. Add the chicken, cashews, and ginger to the cooking garlic. Cook, stirring frequently, until the outside of the chicken has cooked.

7. Stir in the chicken broth, soy sauce, and maple syrup. Add the onion back to the pan and cook, stirring gently, for about 5 minutes.

8. Add the thawed edamame and cook for another 5 to 8 minutes, until the chicken is cooked through. Serve over the cooked brown rice.

Dr. Tim Says . . . If You Have Acid Reflux

Many people who have GERD (gastroesophageal reflux disease) will experience symptoms when eating onions that are cooked lightly or are raw. If you cook the onions for a long time, until they are milky and translucent, they will often be easier to tolerate.

If you have GERD, it's also important to use as little fat when cooking as possible. Many people have trouble with Asian food triggering reflux because it usually has a lot of fat. A recipe like this could have as much as 80 grams of fat per serving in an Asian restaurant! Cutting the fat out is easy, and if you use this recipe as a guide, many of your other Asian favorites can be made GERD friendly.

Ginger and ginger extracts have been shown in many studies to help with nausea and may help prevent reflux.

Day 10 Alternative Dinner Choices

CONVENIENCE MEALS

Lean Cuisine Chicken in Peanut Sauce

RESTAURANT MEALS

Red Lobster Shrimp Cocktail Appetizer with a Side Salad and Baked Potato

Can fat be good for you?

Yes.

It's taken over two decades of controversy, but research has clearly proven just how good fat is for you. As with everything you choose to eat, it is the quality of the fat that's important. We've come to know that unsaturated fats, especially monounsaturated fats such as omega-3 fatty acid, actually help prevent disease, whereas saturated fats should be consumed in moderation and trans fats eliminated from your diet completely (more on these in the next chapter).

There's good reason to be confused, however. Over the last three decades, there have been dozens of competing theories. The low-fat wave of the 1990s, while well-intentioned, wasn't completely correct. At the time, it was known that eating foods high in saturated fat was a health issue, but the message ended up being that all fats were bad. Researchers told us to go fat-free, and it became clear pretty quickly that they had made a mistake. Unfortunately the message in people's minds remained: "All fat is bad."

Fatty acids come in a number of forms and some are critical for your body to function. One of their main roles is to provide storage fuel for the body, but they are also involved in absorption of some vitamins, helping to control inflammation, and also in blood clotting. Our body can produce some fats on its own. Others that we have to eat are known as essential fatty acids (EFAs).

The type of fat you consume is what will have the most effect on your health (for better and for worse). The fatty acid molecule is made up of chains of carbon atoms. Each carbon atom in the chain has either one or two hydrogen atoms attached to it. When there are two hydrogen atoms attached to every carbon atom in the string, the fat is referred to as *saturated*. Saturated fats are those that you want to eat less of (more on that on Day 11). Fats that are *unsaturated* (having fewer hydrogen atoms) are better for you, and the EFAs are those you definitely want more of as part of your diet.

Fats do have more calories per gram than carbohydrates or protein (9 calories per gram for fat and 4 calories per gram each for protein and carbs). Reducing the amount of fat you consume can make a big difference in the number of calories you eat—but don't become obsessed with that.

Getting more unsaturated fats, especially *monounsaturated* fats, helps prevent disease. The two monounsaturated fats that you will hear the most about are *omega-6* and *omega-3* fatty acids. These are considered EFAs because our body can't make these fats on its own. Once you eat these fats, your body is able to process them further into a variety of other fats. Omega-3 fats are anti-inflammatory—and inflammation is the basic cause of conditions such as atherosclerosis and cancers.

The studies of omega-3 fats from fish alone are the most compelling, showing that they both prevent and treat disease, and those fish with the highest levels of monounsaturated fats have been shown to be protective.

Most of the omega-6 fats come from vegetable oils in the form of linoleic acid (LA). This is broken down further in the body and eventually becomes arachidonic acid (AA). These fats can actually have the opposite effect of omega-3s by increasing blood pressure and the inflammatory response. It's important to eat a good balance of omega-3 and omega-6 fats (more omega-3 and less omega-6). Much of the higher levels of omega-6 fats in our diet come from the excess of palm, soybean, canola, and sunflower oils used in processed and fried foods. These are good oils (you'll see me using canola oil in recipes); however, too much of a good thing can cause a problem.

Two of the best sources we have for unsaturated fats are nuts and seeds and their oils. While these ingredients have a lot of calories, this is not often an issue (good quality calories = good quality health). During one study, two groups received either as much extra-virgin olive oil or nuts as they wished to add to their regular diet[2] and were encouraged to use these high-fat, high-calorie ingredients as much as they wanted. There was no weight gain with the users of nuts and olive oil, even though they were consuming more calories, proving once again that eating healthy is about the quality of the calories you consume.

Good fats are quality calories and make for good eating. The best part is that there are a lot of great fats to choose from.

Oils/Fats

OLIVE OIL

This is the granddaddy of healthy fats and is well established as being really good for you. I measure all my fats and oils and use them carefully (especially because a lot of folks using Dr. Gourmet recipes are working at losing weight).

Get yourself a good-quality extra-virgin olive oil for making salads, dressings, sauces, and the like. Use less-expensive olive oils for cooking if you are on a budget. I like using an oil sprayer because it lets me easily coat a pan or a food without using a lot of oil.

GRAPESEED OIL

This is as good as and may actually be better for you than olive oil. In some studies, it has been shown to improve cholesterol profiles better than olive oil. Grapeseed oils do not have quite the same range of flavors that you might find in all of the different olive oils on the market, but I love it because of this. I use it when I don't want a lot of bright, fruity flavors in a recipe. It also has a very high smoke point. This is the temperature at which an oil burns, making grapeseed oil a great choice for searing and other high-temperature cooking.

CANOLA OIL

I don't use canola oil as much as I used to because I like grapeseed oil so much. It is, however, a great choice for cooking and baking (and it's less expensive).

NUTS/SEEDS

Take your pick here, from walnuts to almonds to pistachios and beyond. I keep small amounts of nuts on hand for use in a lot of recipes. I generally purchase raw, unsalted nuts and seeds and keep them in tightly closed plastic bags.

FRUITS

Avocados are full of monounsaturated fat. While they are technically a fruit, these lovely guys are a great source of really healthy, great-quality calories.

Olives, like avocados, are also a fruit and chock-full of not just flavor but great-quality monounsaturated fats.

Remember, eating healthy is about eating great food, not eliminating any single group of ingredients just because the foods contain fats (or carbs or protein). The most important thing about eating healthy is the number of overall calories and also the quality of the calories you choose. Eating great-quality fats means eating great-quality calories.

DAY 11 | DINNER

WHITEFISH IN FOIL WITH VEGETABLES AND TOMATO SAUCE AND CAESAR SALAD

Whitefish in Foil with Vegetables and Tomato Sauce

SERVINGS: 2 ▐ **SERVING SIZE:** 4 OUNCES FISH WITH VEGETABLES ▐ **COOKING TIME:** 30 MINUTES

4 spears asparagus
1 can no-salt-added white beans, drained and rinsed
2 (4-ounce) halibut fillets
¼ teaspoon salt
Freshly ground black pepper
1 small carrot, peeled and cut into matchsticks
¼ small green bell pepper, seeded and cut into matchsticks
¼ small red bell pepper, seeded and cut into matchsticks
4 medium-size cremini mushrooms, sliced
4 large basil leaves
4 teaspoons tomato paste
¼ cup dry white wine
4 teaspoons extra-virgin olive oil

This is a fantastic way to cook fish. It is traditionally baked in parchment paper, but for most people the foil is more practical. You can use almost any combination of fish fillet, vegetables, liquid, and herb or spice, along with the olive oil.

Because it is so simple, you can serve it as an easy weeknight meal as well as a weekend dinner party dish. If you are going to serve it at your dinner party, it's more elegant to use the parchment, although the foil works really well on an outdoor grill. You can prepare the foil pouches up to about 4 hours in advance and the parchment 2 hours before cooking.

This recipe can easily be multiplied or halved.

1. Slice the asparagus lengthwise and then cut the spears into quarters (each spear will end up with eight pieces).

2. Preheat the oven to 400°F. Fold one sheet of aluminum foil in half so that it is almost a square (15 by 12 inches). Starting at one end of the folded edge, cut half of a heart shape in such a way that when the foil is opened it is in the shape of a heart. Repeat with a second piece of foil.

3. Place half of the beans on each piece of foil.

4. Rinse the halibut filets in cold water and pat dry. Put the fillets on top of the beans, centering each on one side of each cut heart so that the other side will fold over the top of the fillet easily. Sprinkle ⅛ teaspoon of the salt over each of the fillets. Sprinkle with pepper. Scatter the carrots, red and green pepper, sliced mushrooms, basil, and asparagus over the fish evenly.

5. Mix together the tomato paste and wine. Pour the mixture evenly over the fillets. Drizzle the top of the fillets with the olive oil.

6. Close the foil by rolling the edge inward, starting at the point of the heart and working around to the base.

7. Place the pouches on a cookie sheet and then into the oven. Lower the heat to 375°F and bake for 15 minutes.

8. Transfer each pouch to a plate and let stand for 30 seconds before cutting the pouch open. Some hot steam will escape when the foil is cut (be careful).

Dr. Tim Says . . . Fish and Omega-3 Fats

Here are the approximate amounts of omega-3 fats per 120 g serving (120 g of fish/meat is about the size of a deck of cards and is just over four ounces).

FISH/SEAFOOD	OMEGA-3	FISH/SEAFOOD	OMEGA-3
Sardines	3,000 mg	Shark	500 mg
Atlantic salmon	2,400 mg	Blue mussel (each)	500 mg
Smoked salmon	2000 mg	Squid/scallops/	400 mg
Halibut	2,000 mg	calamari	
Tuna	1,200 mg	Crayfish	300 mg
Canned salmon	1,000 mg	Canned tuna	290 mg
Oysters (12)	1,000 mg	Grouper	280 mg
Rainbow trout	600 mg	Shrimp (each)	200 mg
Snapper	550 mg	Orange roughy	140 mg

Caesar Salad

SERVINGS: 8 ▌ **SERVING SIZE:** 1 SIDE SALAD ▌ THIS RECIPE CAN EASILY BE DOUBLED ▌
COOKING TIME: 15 MINUTES ▌ THE DRESSING KEEPS WELL TIGHTLY SEALED IN THE RE-
FRIGERATOR FOR 5 TO 7 DAYS

2 cloves garlic, minced
2 anchovy fillets
¼ teaspoon freshly ground
   black pepper
2 tablespoons freshly
   squeezed lemon juice
2 tablespoons Dijon
   mustard
2 tablespoons honey
1½ ounces Parmigiano-
   Reggiano, grated
½ cup nonfat yogurt
2 heads romaine lettuce
   (sliced crosswise)
1 cup reduced-fat croutons

NUTRITION FACTS

Serving size 4- to 5-ounce
   salad
Servings 8
Calories 94
Calories from Fat 20
Total Fat 2 g (4%)
Saturated Fat 1 g (5%)
Trans Fat 0 g
Monounsaturated Fat 1 g
Cholesterol 5 mg (2%)
Sodium 219 mg (9%)
Total Carbohydrates 14 g (5%)
Dietary Fiber 4 g (15%)
Sugars 8 g
Protein 6 g
Vitamin A (182%)
Vitamin C (67%)
Calcium (16%)
Iron (10%)

*Parenthetical percentages
refer to % Daily Value.

As I discussed on Day 1, in reference to the Fettuccine Alfredo recipe, I emphasized how certain flavors can help transform a higher-saturated-fat or higher-calorie recipe into one that tastes the same but is better for you. With this recipe, the key flavors are garlic, mustard, anchovies, and Parmesan cheese.

Because Caesar dressing gets its creamy texture from oil and egg, I looked for substitute ingredients that will give a similar mouthfeel. In this case, the combination of honey and yogurt makes for a rich texture.

1. Place the garlic, anchovies, pepper, lemon juice, mustard, honey, cheese, and yogurt in a blender and process until smooth.

2. Chill for at least 2 hours.

3. Rinse the lettuce, drain, and spin dry. Cut crosswise and place in the refrigerator until needed.

4. Toss the dressing with the romaine lettuce and croutons.

> **Chef Tim Says . . . Eat Romaine Lettuce**
>
> From a nutritional standpoint, lettuce is lettuce. Not many calories but some fiber and, depending on the variety, some fantastic vitamins and minerals, including vitamin K, calcium, and a bit of iron.
>
> Even though I like them all, romaine is my favorite lettuce. It's very versatile. The long, crisp leaves with crunchy spines make for perfect salads. Look for larger heads, as the outer leaves are usually tougher and can be bruised. I like to use these for sandwiches and save the delicate light yellow-green leaves at the heart for my best salads.

Day 11 Alternative Dinner Choices

CONVENIENCE MEALS

Lean Cuisine Lemon Pepper Fish or
Lean Cuisine Szechuan Style Stir Fry with Shrimp

RESTAURANT MEALS

Ruby Tuesday Asian Glazed Salmon

DAY 12 | REDUCE YOUR SATURATED FAT AND ELIMINATE TRANS FATS

One of my favorite fat studies[3] looked at 815 senior citizens to evaluate the role diet might play in Alzheimer's disease. Researchers found a clear correlation between diets high in saturated fat and trans fats and the risk of Alzheimer's. Those who ate the most saturated fat and trans fats had almost twice the risk of Alzheimer's dementia.

Interestingly, total fat didn't matter, but eating more fats from vegetable sources appeared to protect those in the study from developing Alzheimer's. Eating a higher proportion of polyunsaturated to saturated fats was also vital to prevention. Eating more unsaturated fats even moderated the risks of eating a higher percentage of trans fats.

Thousands of studies draw similar conclusions—not just about Alzheimer's but also heart disease, diabetes, and cancer. It's not fat that is the issue, it is *the type of fat*.

How much saturated fat is considered healthy? The current recommendations are that you get about 10 percent of your calories from saturated fat (about 17 grams of saturated fat in a 1,500-calorie diet). That has always seemed a bit vague to me, though. In practical terms, think of reducing the amount of saturated fat in your diet by working at eating leaner meats and fewer fried foods, and getting your fats more from vegetable sources rather than from meats.

Here's the lowdown on which fats are best and which to be careful of when stocking your pantry or fridge.

Meats

The leaner the meat, the better. For instance, regular ground beef that is 20 percent fat contains about 9 grams of saturated fat and 284 calories in a 4-ounce serving. 95 percent lean ground beef (5 percent fat) has only 2.5 grams of saturated fat and about 130 fewer calories. When you're buying meat, look for leaner cuts such as top round, lean ground beef, tenderloin, and flank steak.

Look for lower-fat cold cuts for day-to-day use in sandwiches and so forth. In recipes, I do like to use really high-quality cured meats, such as prosciutto. In small amounts, these rich, high-quality ingredients with higher amounts of fat go a long way toward adding a richer flavor to your dishes.

Butter

Real butter (not margarine or a spread) is mostly saturated fat, but for many recipes there's simply no substitute. A teaspoon contains about 2.5 grams of saturated fat, so I use butter sparingly to enrich sauces and in recipes such as mashed potatoes and baked goods. I purchase the best-quality butter I can, because I use so little that it doesn't end up adding that much fat to a recipe.

Dairy

Low-fat dairy means less saturated fat. Whole milk has about 4.5 grams of saturated fat in a cup. The same cup of low-fat milk (1% milk) contains only 1.5 grams. This holds true for other dairy products, such as yogurt, cream cheese, and cottage cheese.

I do use full-fat cheeses in some recipes, but just as with butter, I use them carefully and I use the best-quality cheeses that I can. An ounce of Gruyère cheese has about 5 grams of saturated fat, but the flavor is so intense that for almost any recipe 1½ ounces per serving will give the same flavor as a lot more of a lower-quality cheese. Great-quality Parmigiano-Reggiano and Romano cheeses are the same: a little goes a really long way.

Making the right ingredient choices is all about using the best-quality products you can—the best-quality calories even when they do contain saturated fat.

We now know that saturated fat is one of the culprits behind an increased risk of not just heart disease and stroke, but also some cancers. Trans fats are even more of a problem. This type of fat does occur naturally in small amounts, but most of the trans fats that are found in foods today have been manufactured. Back as long ago as the 1940s, food producers began saturating vegetable oils in a process called hydrogenation. One by-product of the saturation was the creation of trans fats, which provide a longer shelf life, offer better baking properties, and create a slick texture.

The problem is that trans fats have an even stronger link to heart disease than does a naturally saturated fat such as butter. The good news is, through a combination of government and consumer pressure, most manufacturers are moving away from trans fats pretty quickly. One of the most common sources of these trans fats used to be margarine, but for the most part trans fats have now been eliminated from those products.

This is not, however, the case with processed baked goods that have a long shelf life, such as cookies, cakes, and pies. Be sure to check the package carefully, as trans fats now must to be reported in the Nutrition Facts label on all such foods.

Trans fats' effects extend beyond just heart disease. In one study, researchers analyzed women's diets and other factors in relation to their fertility and found that an increase of just 2 percent in the amount of calories they ate in the form of trans-fatty acids, instead of monounsaturated fats (such as those in olive oil), more than doubled a woman's risk of infertility.[4]

The take-home message here is to avoid trans fats (they are definitely bad for you). As far as saturated fats go, limiting your consumption of these is clearly healthier for you.

DAY 12 | DINNER

PHILLY CHEESE STEAK AND WALDORF SALAD

Dr. Tim Says . . . Eat Reduced-Fat Cheeses

Not only is cheese low in saturated fat better for your health, I feel that in a lot of recipes, lower-fat cheeses work better than full-fat versions do. That's because when they melt, there is less chance that they will separate. There's nothing worse than greasy French onion soup.

Just avoid no-fat cheeses. Besides being bland, because they don't have fat, they don't melt well.

Kraft produces a good sharp Cheddar that is 6 grams of fat per ounce; it is marketed under the Cracker Barrel name (regular Cheddar is 9 grams of fat per ounce). It is labeled "made with 2% milk, reduced fat." Jarlsburg brand produces a very good-quality reduced-fat Swiss cheese. It also has about 6 grams of fat per ounce. You can also fairly easily find reduced-fat Monterey Jack cheeses for your Mexican and Southwestern recipes.

Philly Cheese Steak

SERVINGS: 1 | **SERVING SIZE:** 1 SANDWICH | THIS RECIPE CAN EASILY BE MULTIPLIED | **COOKING TIME:** 30 MINUTES

Spray olive oil
½ medium-size onion, peeled and sliced
1 mini baguette (2.5 ounces or less)
1 tablespoon nonfat mayonnaise
2 ounces roasted flank steak or London broil, sliced thinly
½ ounce reduced-fat Swiss cheese, shredded

NUTRITION FACTS

Serving size 1 sandwich
Servings 1
Calories 395
Calories from Fat 123
Total Fat 14 g (21%)
Saturated Fat 4 g (19%)
Trans Fat 0 g
Monounsaturated Fat 3 g
Cholesterol 41 mg (14%)
Sodium 524 mg (22%)
Total Carbohydrates 43 g (14%)
Dietary Fiber 6 g (25%)
Sugars 9 g
Protein 26 g
Vitamin A (1%)
Vitamin C (8%)
Calcium (23%)
Iron (16%)

*Parenthetical percentages refer to % Daily Value.

This recipe is made from Day 9's Flank Steak (page 69) leftovers and should be eaten immediately.

This recipe will work using any flank steak or London broil recipe.

Recipes with flank steak or London broil make for a wonderful, lean, and tasty dinner, but here's the bonus: leftovers like this Philly Cheese Steak. You do have to choose the right cheese to use on your sandwiches. Regular Cheddar cheese contains about 9 grams of fat per ounce. Lower-fat versions are easy to find and full of flavor. Look for cheeses in the range of 4 to 6 grams per ounce.

1. Spray a nonstick pan with olive oil and place over medium-high heat. After the pan is hot, add the onion and lower the heat to medium. Cook the onion slowly until well browned. Set aside.

2. Preheat the oven to broil. Slice the mini baguette lengthwise and place under the broiler with the cut side of the bread facing up. Broil until the inside is lightly browned.

3. Remove the baguette from the oven, spread the mayonnaise on the bread, and top with the sliced flank steak, Top with the onion and then place the Swiss cheese on top of the sandwich.

4. Return the open-faced sandwich to the oven, cheese side up, and broil until the cheese is hot and melted. Serve immediately.

Waldorf Salad

SERVINGS: 8 | **SERVING SIZE:** ¾ CUP | THIS RECIPE KEEPS FAIRLY WELL REFRIGERATED FOR ABOUT 2 DAYS

2 Granny Smith apples, cored and cut into ¼-inch cubes
1 Red Delicious apple, cored and cut into ¼-inch cubes
1 tablespoon freshly squeezed lemon juice
1 cup large-diced celery
¼ cup coarsely chopped walnuts
¼ cup raisins
¼ cup low-fat mayonnaise
¼ cup low-fat sour cream
1½ teaspoons honey

Waldorf salad is one of the ultimate comfort foods for me. There's a great balance of sweet and tart flavors. You don't need the full-fat mayonnaise to get a fantastic creamy texture.

1. Mix the cubed apples with the lemon juice. Add the celery, walnuts, and raisins. Toss.
2. Add the mayonnaise, sour cream, and honey, and gently fold together until well blended.
3. Chill for at least 2 hours before serving.

NUTRITION FACTS

Serving size ¾ cup
Servings 8
Calories 123
Calories from Fat 52
Total Fat 6 g (9%)
Saturated Fat 1 g (6%)
Trans Fat 0 g
Monounsaturated Fat 0 g
Cholesterol 7 mg (2%)
Sodium 75 mg (3%)
Total Carbohydrates 18 g (6%)
Dietary Fiber 2 g (7%)
Sugars 14 g
Protein 1 g
Vitamin A (4%)
Vitamin C (8%)
Calcium (3%)
Iron (2%)

*Parenthetical percentages refer to % Daily Value.

Day 12 Alternative Dinner Choices

CONVENIENCE MEALS

Lean Cuisine Chicken, Spinach, and Mushroom Panini or
Lean Cuisine Southwest-Style Chicken Panini

RESTAURANT MEALS

Panera Bread Half-Serving Chicken Tomesto on French Bread with a Large Fresh Fruit Cup

Dr. Tim Says . . . Eat an Apple a Day
The old adage is true. There's no doubt that apples are good for you. A single apple has all of 70 calories but contains over 3 grams of fiber. Sweet and satisfying, apples are the perfect way to get healthy.

> **Chef Tim Says . . . Cooking with Apples**
>
> For baking, choose Granny Smith apples. This variety is firm enough to hold up to heat and when cooked, a subtle sweetness combines with a tartness that comes through in baked goods. Likewise, using a Granny Smith alongside a sweeter apple in salads is fantastic. The combination of a sweeter Red Delicious apple with the tart Granny Smith for Waldorf salad is a great example.
>
> The texture of Roma apples makes them a great choice for cooking, but they have a creamier sweetness and lack the tartness of the Granny Smith.
>
> Red Delicious apples don't hold up as well to cooking. I love the crunchy texture and sweetness for snacking and for salads, however. The same holds true for Gala and Jonagold apples. They're not as good a choice for baking, but they're great for snacking.
>
> Golden Delicious makes for a good all-purpose apple to have on hand. They are great for snacking and for salads, but do hold up well to baking. Interestingly, the flesh of the Golden Delicious will not oxidize as fast and remains white longer than does other varieties in recipes such as salads.

DAY 13 | CARBS ARE GOOD FOR YOU, TOO

Every time I hear someone say that carbs are bad for you, I just want to scream—just go outside and start hollering as loud as I can. It's just crazy.

Take this as gospel: *Carbohydrates are good for you!*

Your body needs carbs. They are the fuel that it uses to get you through the day on a minute-by-minute basis.

What exactly is a carb? Carbohydrates are chains of sugar molecules called *saccharides*. A single sugar molecule is known as a *monosaccharide*, whereas two sugars joined together are called a *disaccharide*. These latter are called *simple sugars* because they easily break down in the body into monosaccharides. The monosaccharide glucose is important because it's the primary fuel for your body and all usable carbohydrates contain glucose molecules. Combining the monosaccharides glucose and fructose results in the disaccharide called *sucrose* (good old-fashioned table sugar).

Chains longer than two monosacchrides are called *polysaccharides*. These are considered complex carbohydrates (also called *starches* or *complex sugars*). Starches contain at least some glucose. These complex carbohydrates break down more slowly than simple carbs. Research shows that eating a diet that is high in more complex carbohydrates helps you lose weight more easily. There are a number of reasons for this, including that the complex carbs in such foods as whole wheat pasta, beans, and oatmeal are more filling and by breaking down slower help you feel satisfied longer. This may also be because they don't cause as dramatic a surge in insulin and other hormones.

When you look at the Nutrition Facts label on food packaging, you'll see Total Carbohydrates listed in grams. This is the total amount of carbs—both simple and complex. Sugars are listed for the amount of simple carbohydrates. Subtract the simple carbs from the total carbs and you have about the number of grams of complex carbohydrates, or starches. When you look at a Nutrition Facts label (more about this on Day 15), you should try to keep the grams of sugar as low as possible (under 6 grams per serving) and the fiber as high as possible.

None of this sounds particularly evil, but like fats, carbohydrates have come to be feared as the culprit responsible for weight gain. This is just plain silly. Although there is evidence that people do lose weight on Atkins-type low-carb diets, they are not the miracle diets that they are made out to be.

The reason that low-carb diets work is because of the poor-quality carbohydrate choices people generally make. It's easy to lose weight when you just stop eating potato chips, French fries, crackers, candy, cake, ice cream, and so on. This is why people succeed on the Atkins or South Beach diet: They simply quit eating junk. This is a good thing and, as you will hear me say over and over, weight loss is about eating fewer calories than you burn. That said, eating a balance of calories—good carbohydrates, protein, healthy fats—is what helps you stay slim. However, most folks can't sustain their weight loss on such fad diets because the diets are too limiting.

To eat healthy and lose weight, you do not have to quit eating carbs altogether. Just make better carb choices. Again, choose the best-quality calories. For instance, if you are going to have pasta, choose whole wheat pasta. The higher fiber will keep you satisfied longer. The same holds true for such things as brown rice instead of white and yams instead of potatoes.

These more complex, higher-fiber carbohydrates have been shown, time and again, to be better for you.

The clichéd example is candy vs. a piece of fruit. There's very strong research showing that you will actually be more satisfied and feel better about yourself by eating the apple. For instance, a Milky Way Bar has 240 calories. The candy has 41 grams of carbohydrates, of which 35 grams are sugar (remember the rule of thumb for sugar: 4 grams = 1 teaspoon). That works out to about 9 teaspoons of sugar (rather a lot). As with many low-quality calorie foods, there's also a lot of fat: 10 grams of fat per bar, including 7 grams of saturated fat. Open the candy bar, eat it in a few minutes, it's full of sugar (and fat), and it's gone. Because it's not very complex, you aren't as satisfied and you're left still craving more food.

Compare this to having a large apple: fewer calories (116) and fewer carbs (30) but without any fat. It's full of fiber, filling, and really satisfying. There's sugar in the apple but a better balance of sugars. The total sugar content is only around 7 teaspoons, but of that, only 1 teaspoon is table sugar and the rest is natural fruit sugars. Interestingly, there's also good research showing that folks are just as satisfied eating an apple as when they eat chocolate, but they don't feel as guilty about eating the apple as they do about eating the chocolate.[5]

Whatever carbohydrate you choose, the most important thing is to know what constitutes the right portion size. Simply knowing what the best choices are and how much is in a serving means that you can have your carbs and eat them, too. Review the good carbohydrate choices from Day 3 and there will be more to come on Day 35. If you forget, remember brown is good—brown pasta, brown bread, brown rice, oatmeal, yams, sweet potatoes—and fruit is really good for you.

Salmon-Squash Risotto

SERVINGS: 2 ▌ **SERVING SIZE:** ABOUT 2 CUPS ▌ THIS RECIPE CAN EASILY BE MULTIPLIED ▌ **COOKING TIME:** 30 MINUTES

1 pound yellow summer squash, seeded and cut into ½-inch dice
Spray olive oil
1 teaspoon extra-virgin olive oil
1 clove garlic, minced
1 medium-size onion, diced
2 tablespoons pumpkin seeds
½ cup uncooked arborio rice
½ cup no-salt-added chicken stock
⅛ teaspoon salt
6 ounces salmon fillet, skin removed, cut into small strips
1 tablespoon fresh oregano
1 ounce Parmigiano-Reggiano, grated
Freshly ground black pepper

NUTRITION FACTS

Serving size about 2 cups
Servings 2
Calories 524
Calories from Fat 161
Total Fat 18 g (28%)
Saturated Fat 5 g (25%)
Trans Fat 0 g
Monounsaturated Fat 8 g
Cholesterol 62 mg (21%)
Sodium 437 mg (18%)
Total Carbohydrates 58 g (19%)
Dietary Fiber 7 g (29%)
Sugars 3 g
Protein 33 g
Vitamin A (12%)
Vitamin C (41%)
Calcium (25%)
Iron (31%)

*Parenthetical percentages refer to % Daily Value.

This keeps well for about 48 hours in the fridge. Leftover salmon can still be tasty as long as it is cooked carefully to begin with. By cooking the salmon gently at the end of this recipe, it won't be overcooked when the leftovers are reheated. Reheat the leftover risotto very gently, by heating on medium heat in the microwave for 90 seconds. Stir gently and heat for another 90 to 120 seconds until hot.

This recipe is about as close to the Mediterranean diet as you can get, yet it is really appealing to American tastes. It's all there and all familiar— rice, squash, pumpkin seeds, cheese, salmon, olive oil—and it's all great tasting. As you'll see in later chapters, it has ingredients from six categories of the Mediterranean diet.

1. Place a large ovenproof nonstick skillet in the oven and preheat to 375°F. When the pan is hot, add the diced squash and spray lightly with olive oil. Toss and return the pan to the oven. About every 7 minutes, remove the pan and toss the squash carefully. After about 20 minutes, the squash cubes should be lightly browned.

2. While the squash is cooking, heat the teaspoon of olive oil over medium heat in a medium-size stockpot. Add the garlic and cook slowly. Do not allow to brown.

3. When the garlic is soft and translucent, add the onion and pumpkin seeds and cook until the onion is translucent. Add the rice and cook for about 2 minutes, stirring frequently.

4. Lower the heat to medium and add the chicken stock. Stir well. Cook for 1 minute and add 2 cups of water, then the salt.

5. Cook over medium-heat, stirring occasionally so that the rice will not stick to the bottom. After about 15 minutes, check to see if the rice is done. Add more water, ¼ cup at a time, as needed.

6. Add the salmon strips and oregano when the rice is soft but not mushy. Cook for about 3 minutes and add the roasted squash and the Parmesan. Stir and cook for another minute over very low heat. Season with pepper to taste and serve.

Day 13 Alternative Dinner Choices

CONVENIENCE MEALS

Lean Cuisine Szechuan Style Stir Fry with Shrimp

RESTAURANT MEALS

Panera Boston Clam Chowder with a Large Fresh Fruit Cup

Chef Tim Says . . . Eat Arborio Rice

Arborio is a slightly round, short-grain rice with a high starch content. The grains have a pearly sheen. Although white rice might not be as good for you as brown rice, that doesn't mean that you can't have it, too. Risottos made with arborio rice are healthy because as arborio rice cooks, its starch is released into the cooking liquid to make a creamy, rich sauce. As such, you don't need to add high-calorie ingredients such as butter or cream to make a rich, delicious dish.

The rice is grown widely in Europe, especially in Italy, but also in Spain (where Calasparra rice is more commonly used). There are now many growers in the United States that produce an excellent-quality arborio rice.

The term *risotto* technically refers to the Italian rice dish made with arborio rice, although the two terms have become nearly synonymous.

Fiber is what your grandma used to call "roughage." It's not one particular food, but it's simply the part of foods that your body can't digest. Fiber is technically carbohydrates, but your body doesn't have the enzymes to break fiber down as it does sucrose. As a result, the fiber is not absorbed and essentially has no calories. So why should you care? Fiber helps prevent cancer and lowers the risk of heart disease, plus high-fiber diets have been shown to reduce cholesterol levels and help diabetics control their blood sugars. Every week, there's another study showing how important it is to get more fiber in your diet.

In one study, researchers looked at the relationship between eating whole grains, refined grains, or cereal fiber and the risk factors for heart disease, high cholesterol, and diabetes.[6] Those with the highest intake of these foods had a lower BMI, weight, and waist circumference. They also had better cholesterol scores and a normal score in a two-hour insulin reaction test (a common test for diabetes and prediabetic conditions).

Eating fiber also helps you maintain a healthy weight. One of my favorite pieces of research (on any topic) showed that those who ate a high-fiber breakfast were more satisfied through the morning, ate less lunch, and had improved blood sugar levels later in the day.[7] Researchers in Spain looked at a large-scale, five-year study of nutrition. They found that for men, higher fiber intake meant a lower risk of weight gain: up to 48 percent lower for the highest intake of fiber. For women, those eating the most fiber had a decreased risk of weight gain of 19 percent.

Fiber comes in two forms: soluble and insoluble. *Soluble fiber* is thought of as "sticky" fiber and is more effective in lowering cholesterol. It is found in beans and some grains, such as oat bran, oatmeal, and rye. Almost all fruits, such as apples, grapes, peaches, oranges, and pears, are high in soluble fiber (think sticky fruits). Most vegetables are also high in soluble fiber. *Insoluble fiber* is found in whole-grain products such as whole wheat flour and whole-grain breads and pastas, as well as in cereal grains such as rice, wild rice, and seeds.

Most of us need to increase the amount of fiber in our diet by at least double. The average American gets only 10 to 15 grams of fiber per day, whereas 25 to 30 grams per day are optimum. There are simple changes you can make that will put more fiber in your life.

For breakfast, choose whole-grain cereals such as shredded wheat, bran flakes, 100% bran, and oatmeal. Take a moment in the grocery store to look at the box and compare the amounts of fiber in these cereals with the one you are eating. Look carefully, because many cereals will have higher fiber but will sometimes contain a lot of sugar as well.

If you like toast for breakfast, choose breads with higher fiber. Most breads will have only about 2 grams per slice, but it's easy to find choices with up to 5 grams. Even if the label says "whole wheat," you may find that it doesn't have much fiber. Check the label, as many manufacturers of breads and cereals use the term "whole-grain flour" when the flour is, in fact, not whole wheat. Use the same high-fiber breads for your sandwiches at lunch.

Simply substituting ingredients in your favorite dinner recipes can help you get more fiber. Use whole wheat pastas, and choose brown rice or wild rice in place of white rice. Replace potatoes with sweet potatoes or yams. Choose recipes that contain beans and other legumes such as lentils and split peas.

Snacking on fruit is a great way to get more fiber. Fruits that are good high-fiber choices are apples, strawberries, and raisins.

And it's never too late to put more fiber in your diet. One study[8] of people over age sixty-five showed that those who consumed the highest level of cereal fiber (as opposed to vegetable or fruit fiber) had a 21 percent lower risk of heart disease than did those who ate the least cereal fiber. This is quite possibly the easiest change you can make in your diet.

DAY 14 | DINNER

LEFTOVER SALMON-SQUASH RISOTTO (PAGE 92)

Day 14 Alternative Meals

Lean Cuisine Salmon with Basil

Red Lobster Grilled Fish

CHAPTER 3 | *WEEK 3 GOALS*

Following this plan, you will lose weight more slowly than on other plans you may have tried, but keep in mind this is about *sustained* weight loss. The first three weeks lay the foundation for your long-term success.

In the third week, you'll learn how to read and use food labels to your advantage. There's a lot of information on food packaging, including those you have already learned about: calories, fats, carbohydrates, and cholesterol. One of the most important is salt, and this week you'll find out why we doctors believe you should move toward limiting your sodium intake.

In the second half of the week, you'll begin learning about menu planning and one of the most important skills of all, knowing portion size.

At the end of the week, we'll discuss cleaning out your pantry and getting rid of as many processed foods as possible.

This week is full of great comfort food standards, including Sloppy Joes, taco salad, pizza, and chili.

This week, you'll:

▊ Learn how to read a food label
▊ Understand the importance of salt and sodium in diet and health
▊ Learn about dietary cholesterol

- Begin measuring your food to help you understand portion size better
- Learn about the right portion sizes
- Clean out your pantry

WEEK 3 | MENU

A personalized shopping list for Week 3 can be found at DrGourmet.com/shoppinglist.

DAY 15 | READ EVERY FOOD LABEL CAREFULLY

When I first started writing about food and nutrition, there wasn't much information available. At the time, the government didn't require that manufacturers list nutrition information on their packages. Now we have all this extra information. I think that sometimes all that data overwhelms people and they end up ignoring the label, but it is critical that you know how to use the Nutrition Facts box—and what really matters on it. Understanding a small amount of very simple information can help you easily lose a lot of weight.

A good example is a 16-ounce bottle of orange juice—a healthy choice, right? A quick glance at the Nutrition Facts shows that there are only 120 calories per serving, but if you don't look closely you might not notice that there are two servings in the bottle. That's really 240 calories! Drinking 240 extra calories per day equals about ½ pound of weight gain each week (or ½ pound of weight loss by not drinking the orange juice).

Look at the Nutrition Facts in separate sections—it makes it easier to use. The first section (in gray) shows you the serving size and the number of servings in the package. As with the orange juice example, it's easy to get tripped up here. In the real world, those smaller packages are what you'd customarily eat as single servings (who's going to eat only one of the two

WEEK 3 MENU

RECIPE	CONVENIENCE FOOD ALTERNATIVE	RESTAURANT MEAL ALTERNATIVE
DAY 15		
Sloppy Joes and Salad with Thousand Island Dressing	Michael Angelo's Lasagna with Meat Sauce with a Side Salad	Wendy's Chili with Spring Mix Salad
DAY 16		
Black Bean and Corn Taco Salad	Lean Cuisine Linguine Carbonara	P. F. Chang's Steamed Buddha's Feast with Vegetarian Lettuce Wraps
DAY 17		
Pizza with Thai Peanut Sauce and Scallops	Wolfgang Puck's Grilled Vegetable Cheeseless Pizza	Pizza Hut Half-Serving Cheese Only Personal Pan Pizza
DAY 18		
White Bean Chili and Salad with Thousand Island Dressing	Kashi Southwest Style Chicken	Ruby Tuesday White Bean Chicken Chili with Side Salad
DAY 19		
Grouper with White Beans and Tomato Vinaigrette	Michael Angelo's Italian Natural Cuisine Vegetable Lasagna	Red Lobster Grilled Halibut or Red Lobster Garlic-Grilled Jumbo Shrimp
DAY 20		
Leftover White Bean Chili and Parmesan Squash	Kashi Southwest Style Chicken	Ruby Tuesday White Bean Chicken Chili with Side Salad
DAY 21		
Pumpkin-Crusted Trout with Lemon Sauce, Wild Rice, and Roasted Tomatoes	Lean Cuisine Szechuan Style Stir Fry with Shrimp Lean Cuisine Lemon Pepper Fish	Red Lobster Garlic-Grilled Jumbo Shrimp or Red Lobster Grilled Fish

Nutrition Facts

Serving Size 1 cup (228g)
Servings Per Container 2

Amount Per Serving

Calories 250   Calories from Fat 110

	% Daily Value*
Total Fat 12g	18%
Saturated Fat 3g	15%
Trans Fat 3g	
Cholesterol 30mg	10%
Sodium 470mg	20%
Total Carbohydrate 31g	10%
Dietary Fiber 0g	0%
Sugars 5g	
Protein 5g	

Vitamin A	4%
Vitamin C	2%
Calcium	20%
Iron	4%

*Percent Daily Values are based on a 2,000 calorie diet. Your Daily Values may be higher or lower depending on your calorie needs.

*Percent Daily Values are based on a 2,000 calorie diet. Your Daily Values may be higher or lower depending on your calorie needs.

	Calories	2,000	2,500
Total fat	Less than	65g	80g
Sat fat	Less than	20g	25g
Cholesterol	Less than	300mg	300mg
Sodium	Less than	2,400mg	2,400mg
Total Carbohydrate		300g	375g
Dietary Fiber		25g	30g

1. Always start by looking at the serving size and the number of servings in the package.

2. The next section shows the number of calories per serving. Simple enough, but again, how many servings are in the container?

This section also tells you how many of those calories are from fat. Divide this number by total calories. Nearly half the calories are from fat. In our example, that's a lot. A good rule of thumb is that a complete meal should have fewer than one-third of its calories from fat. Keep in mind that some ingredients, such as olive oil, are all fat, but as we discussed on Day 11, some fats are good for you.

3. Section three is the most important, showing you the amount of fat, cholesterol, and sodium in each serving. There is also a breakdown of the fats by type: saturated and trans fats. If the food contains any trans fat, don't buy it. Your foods or ingredients should have zero (0) grams trans fats.

4. Carbohydrates, dietary fiber (the more, the better), and proteins are in the next section. Look closely at the amount of sugars in your foods. While a lot of foods, such as fruits and juices, are high in natural sugars, it's a good idea to limit the amount of added sugars. Each teaspoon of sugar is 5 grams of carbohydrate, so when you're looking at an item with added sugar, simply multiply the number of grams of sugar by 4 to know how many added calories you are getting.

5. The fifth section shows you information on vitamins and minerals. Vitamins and minerals are reported at the percent of Recommended Daily Allowance, so generally speaking, the higher the better.

6. The numbers along the right side of the above items should be used as a guide for quick and easy information. They show the "Percent Daily Value" for fat, cholesterol, sodium, etc. that you should have in a day. This food has 18 percent, or about one-fifth of the amount of fat you should consume for the day.

Keep in mind that these percentages are based on a 2,000-calorie-per-day diet. If you are eating 1,500 calories per day, that's 75 percent of 2,000 calories, and the daily value needs to adjust accordingly. You will also need to adjust if you are eating more calories.

7. The last section is a guide to the recommended amounts of fats, cholesterol, sodium, etc. The requirement is to report on 2,000 and 2,500 calories. Not many people should be eating 2,000 or more calories per day, however. Here's the information for a 1,500 calorie diet:

Total Fat: Less than 49 grams
Sat. Fat: Less than 15 grams
Cholesterol: Less than 300 mg
Sodium: Less than 2,400mg
Total Carbohydrate: Less than 225 grams
Dietary Fiber: 20 grams

cookies in the package that comes out of the vending machine?), but manufacturers will list them as two or three servings. Take a look at the next small bag of potato chips you run across. How many servings are in it?

Use the 20/5 Rule

You can use the percentages along the right side of the Nutrition Facts box to your advantage. A quick and easy way to evaluate a food is the 20/5 rule. When you look at a package, if the *fat, sodium,* or *cholesterol* are less than 5 percent of the Daily Value, that's a good sign. If any are over 20 percent, reconsider. For *total carbohydrates, dietary fiber, vitamins,* and *minerals,* 5 percent or less of the Daily Value is not good; 20 percent or higher is good.

Here's a table to help:

Keep in mind that this rule works better for foods you might purchase ready made, such as snacks, prepared foods, and convenience foods. As such, there are exceptions: whole, unprocessed foods will be naturally high in one macronutrient or another. Butter, for example, is not inherently bad for you, even though it is almost all fat. Choosing your foods and ingredients is about balance. An ingredient such as soy sauce, for example, will be high in sodium by this measure (even the low-salt versions) but as an ingredient that's okay. However, a serving of frozen pizza that contains

20/5 RULE		
	LESS THAN 5% DAILY VALUE	MORE THAN 20% DAILY VALUE
Fat	Good	May not be as good
Sodium	Good	May not be as good
Cholesterol	Good	May not be as good
Carbohydrates	May not be as good	Good
Fiber	May not be as good	Good
Vitamins A and C	May not be as good	Good
Calcium and Iron	May not be as good	Good

50 percent of the total sodium you need for a day is not such a great idea. This guideline can work when you are looking at recipes in magazines or cookbooks that list nutrition information, but again, it is a guideline. One recipe might be over 20 percent of the Daily Value for fat, for instance, but might serve as a complete meal and be okay.

Now test yourself using the Nutrition Facts guide and a few cans or boxes from your pantry. Then you'll be primed to make better choices the next time you go to the grocery store.

Check the Ingredient List

Another good guide can be looking at the ingredients printed on the label. They must be listed in order of amount by weight. If the first three ingredients contain any of the following, you might want to take a second look at the Nutrition Facts label.

Salt
Monosodium glutamate (MSG)
Hydrolyzed vegetable protein (this is essentially MSG)
Free glutamate
Yeast extract or autolyzed yeast
Sodium nitrate or sodium nitrite
Lard
Hydrogenated oil
Palm oil or palm kernel oil
Vegetable shortening
Sugars
High-fructose corn syrup

IF THE LABEL SAYS . . .

Diet: For a product to be labeled "diet" it must either be low calorie, reduced calorie, or have a special use in a diet. Diabetic foods could be labeled "diet" for this reason.

More: "More" means that a serving of food must contain a nutrient that is at least 10 percent more of the Daily Value than the reference food. This applies to all foods, whether they have been altered in some way or not. For example, "more" could be used when a food manufacturer might use a grain with more fiber in a cereal. If the cereal has 10 percent more fiber than does a regular cereal, the package could be labeled "more fiber."

Foods labeled "fortified," "enriched," "added," "extra," and "plus" are similar, but in these cases the food must be one that has been altered. The example here would be a cereal that has simply had fiber added to it to increase the fiber content, instead of using a different grain already containing that fiber.

Less: Foods labeled "less" must contain 25 percent less of a particular nutrient or 25 percent fewer calories than a similar food. This applies to foods whether they have been altered or not. Pretzels, for example, which have 25 percent less fat than potato chips are allowed to use the "less" claim. "Fewer" means the same thing as "less."

High: If the word "high" is used on the label, the product must have at least 20 percent or more of the Daily Value for a particular nutrient in a serving. So if a container says "high fiber," the food must have at least 5 grams of fiber in a serving.

Good source: The term "good source" on a label is similar to the term "high," but the food only has to have between 10 and 19 percent of the Daily Value for a particular nutrient.

DAY 15 | DINNER

SLOPPY JOES AND SALAD WITH THOUSAND ISLAND DRESSING

Sloppy Joes

SERVINGS: 4 ▌ **SERVING SIZE:** ABOUT 1½ CUPS SLOPPY JOE ON A BUN ▌ THIS RECIPE
CAN EASILY BE MULTIPLIED ▌ **COOKING TIME:** 30 MINUTES ▌ THIS RECIPE MAKES GREAT
LEFTOVERS. REHEAT GENTLY.

1 teaspoon olive oil
1 large onion, diced
1 rib celery, diced
1 large carrot, peeled and
    diced
1 small green bell pepper,
    seeded and diced
1 pound 97% lean ground
    beef
1 tablespoon red wine
    vinegar
1 tablespoon Worcestershire
    sauce
½ teaspoon paprika
2 tablespoons tomato paste
Freshly ground black
    pepper
4 whole wheat hamburger
    buns or kaiser rolls

NUTRITION FACTS

Serving size about 1½ cups
    Sloppy Joe on a bun
Servings 4
Calories 340
Calories from Fat 71
Total Fat 8 g (12%)
Saturated Fat 3 g (15%)
Trans Fat 0 g
Monounsaturated Fat 3 g
Cholesterol 69 mg (23%)
Sodium 453 mg (19%)
Total Carbohydrates 39 g (13%)
Dietary Fiber 7 g (26%)
Sugars 12 g
Protein 30 g
Vitamin A (68%)
Vitamin C (46%)
Calcium (11%)
Iron (27%)

*Parenthetical percentages
refer to % Daily Value.

I love Sloppy Joes, one of those comfort foods that's cheap, easy to make, and can really be good for you. A lot of recipes for Sloppy Joes have poor-quality calories—too much saturated fat and a ton of salt. But just a few tweaks can help you go from lousy calorie to quality calorie.

Rather than getting your Sloppy Joe out of a can or a seasoning packet, choose lean ground beef, fresh veggies, and these simple spices. Lower in fat and salt, and with a fresh, homemade taste, this recipe won't take much longer than the "instant" mixes. Using whole wheat hamburger buns will usually double (and sometimes triple) the amount of fiber.

1. Place the olive oil in a large skillet over medium-high heat. Add the onion, celery, carrot, and bell pepper. Cook for about 5 minutes, stirring occasionally.

2. Add the ground beef and cook, stirring frequently, until it is browned.

3. Add the vinegar, Worcestershire, paprika, tomato paste, ground pepper to taste, and 1½ cups of water. Lower the heat to medium-low and simmer for about 20 minutes, stirring occasionally.

4. Serve over lightly toasted hamburger buns.

Salad with Thousand Island Dressing

SERVINGS: 6 ▌ **SERVING SIZE:** ¼ CUP ▌ THIS RECIPE CAN EASILY BE DOUBLED OR TRIPLED ▌ **COOKING TIME:** 15 MINUTES

1 large egg
½ cup nonfat mayonnaise
½ cup nonfat yogurt
¼ cup no-salt-added ketchup
2 tablespoons sweet pickle relish
1 tablespoon minced shallot
3 tablespoons diced celery
⅛ teaspoon freshly ground black pepper
⅛ teaspoon salt

NUTRITION FACTS

Serving size ¼ cup
Servings 6
Calories 57
Calories from Fat 14
Total Fat 2 g (2%)
Saturated Fat 0 g (0%)
Trans Fat 0 g
Monounsaturated Fat 0 g
Cholesterol 38 mg (13%)
Sodium 282 mg (12%)
Total Carbohydrates 9 g (3%)
Dietary Fiber 1 g (2%)
Sugars 6 g
Protein 3 g
Vitamin A (5%)
Vitamin C (3%)
Calcium (5%)
Iron (27%)

*Parenthetical percentages refer to % Daily Value.

Pair this dressing with your favorite salad greens.

The hard-boiled egg adds so much to this recipe. While it adds some fat and calories, it's a minimal amount. The cooked egg yolk adds creaminess to the dressing and the egg white provides the all-important islands. (What? You didn't think there were supposed to be islands in Thousand Island dressing?) Best of all, a bottled dressing is 130 calories or more for 2 tablespoons, whereas this one has only 57 calories.

This recipe keeps well for 4 to 5 days in the refrigerator.

1. Place 4 cups of water in a small pan over high heat. When the water is boiling, place the egg (in the shell) gently in the pan (be careful not to crack it) and cook at a boil for 3 minutes. Turn off the heat and let the egg stand in the hot water for 12 minutes.

2. Remove the egg from the hot water and let stand on the counter while mixing the other ingredients.

3. Stir the mayonnaise, yogurt, ketchup, pickle relish, shallot, celery, pepper, and salt together in a small mixing bowl.

4. Crack the eggshell and then run under cool water. Peel the hard-boiled egg and then chop coarsely. Add it to the dressing and stir well.

5. Place the dressing in a storage container and refrigerate for at least an hour before serving.

Myth: Celery is "Negative Calories."

Truth: It is true that celery has almost no calories. A medium-size stalk contains all of 6 calories. It's also pretty good for you in that a large stalk has about a gram of fiber and is high in calcium and trace minerals. Interestingly, celery is also fairly high in sodium, for a vegetable, at 50 mg for a large stalk.

The theory that many people put forward is that your body uses more than 6 calories to chew and digest the celery. There are actually books written about the negative calorie concept but there's no reliable research to support the claim.

The body uses between 10 and 15 percent of the calories you consume for the total process of digestion. In someone consuming 1,500 calories per day, that's 225 calories in 24 hours. It takes the same 225 calories for digestion, whether you eat those 1,500 calories per day as celery or as bread. The difference is that you would have to eat 250 stalks of celery per day to eat 1,500 calories, as opposed to about fifteen slices of bread.

Here's how celery can help people lose weight: It tastes good, it takes time to chew, it's filling, and it's low in calories.

Day 15 Alternative Dinner Choices

CONVENIENCE MEALS

Michael Angelo's Lasagna with Meat Sauce with a Side Salad

RESTAURANT MEALS

Wendy's Chili with Spring Mix Salad

DAY 16 | *HOLD THE SALT*

We eat too much salt. It might be hard to believe, but the average person eats more than 6,000 milligrams (mg) of sodium every day. That works out to about 2½ teaspoons of salt, which is about 2½ times the recommended amount of 2,400 mg per day.

The main issue with consuming too much salt is that it has a clear effect on blood pressure. One major study showed that the more salt consumed by participants, the greater increase in their blood pressure over time. Conversely, in studies that limit sodium intake, there is a dramatic decrease in blood pressure. Most dramatically, study participants who consume a high-sodium diet of 6 grams per day vs. those on a 1,500 mg sodium restricted diet increased their risk of death from heart disease by over 50 percent.[1]

It appears that a low-sodium diet may help control weight. In a study of different cultures around the world, those consuming the lowest-sodium diets had the lowest BMI.[2] In our own culture, salt consumption is a profound problem. Research estimates that reducing salt intake could save 150,000 lives each year. That's a lot of our relatives, friends, and co-workers.

If you are used to eating a lot of salt, the good news is that your taste buds can learn to do without all that sodium. A great study[3] placed a group of people on a sodium-restricted diet for five months. Their subjective response to the saltiness in solutions, soups, and crackers was measured before, during, and after the diet. The same measurements were made in a control group that continued their usual diet. In the group that ate less salt, the perceived intensity of salt in crackers increased over the five-month period. In other words, the same crackers seemed to taste more and more salty as the study progressed. The amount of added salt that was required for food to taste its best fell in the study group but not in the control group.

Here's how to make the change and reduce the amount of salt in your diet:

Step One: That 2,400 mg of salt per day recommendation is a total of 1 teaspoon of salt per day *total*. If you measure your salt when you cook instead of throwing it in willy-nilly, you'll find that eating less sodium is pretty easy. It's a simple step to being healthier.

Step Two: Most frozen foods, convenience meals, fast food, and quick snacks have a lot of added sodium. Make fresh meals as often as possible. Start slowly, and each week plan to make more home-made meals part of your diet. Remember that leftovers of freshly made meals count as fresh meals as well.

Step Three: Don't buy or eat processed foods. Those boxed foods, such as macaroni and cheese or hamburger extenders, have tons of added sodium. Once again, cook it fresh. Cooking food from scratch takes a bit more time, but it tastes better and is better for you. When you cook your own meals, you control the amount of salt in your diet.

Step Four: If you must buy a processed food, look at the amount of salt on the label. The sodium content is the one item on the Nutrition Facts label that is pretty straightforward. This is a great place to use the 20/5 guideline.

Look carefully at processed foods that claim to be reduced/low fat, as the manufacturer will often add sugar or salt to replace the texture or flavor that might be lost in lowering the fat content.

Cutting out the added salt in your diet is one of the simplest ways to make a major change in your health. Make changes gradually and your taste buds will learn to appreciate the true flavors of your food. Not only will your food taste better, you'll be so much healthier for it.

Black Bean and Corn Taco Salad

SERVINGS: 2 ▌ **SERVING SIZE:** 1 LARGE SALAD ▌ THIS RECIPE CAN EASILY BE DOUBLED OR TRIPLED ▌ **COOKING TIME:** 30 MINUTES ▌ THE COOKED CHICKEN WILL KEEP WELL IN THE REFRIGERATOR FOR ABOUT 2 DAYS

Spray oil
1 medium-size onion, diced
8 ounces boneless, skinless chicken breast, cut into small dice
½ teaspoon chili powder
⅛ teaspoon cayenne
⅛ teaspoon salt
2 ounces low-fat tortilla chips
3 cups iceberg lettuce, sliced thinly
½ cup canned no-salt black beans, drained and rinsed
1 large tomato, sliced into small wedges
2 tablespoons dried pumpkin seeds
1 green onion, sliced
2 ounces reduced-fat Monterey Jack cheese, shredded
2 tablespoons reduced-fat sour cream
6 tablespoons Tomatillo Salsa (recipe follows) or other reduced-sodium salsa

Who would have thought that taco salad could be so good for you? This version is relatively low in fat, low in sodium, and high in fiber. There's also a lot of vitamin A and C as well as iron and calcium.

Choose lower-fat, low-sodium tortilla chips and make sure that they are trans fat free.

This recipe is best with Tomatillo Salsa (recipe follows). If you don't have time to make the Tomatillo Salsa, look for a ready-made salsa that is lower in salt. Most of the major brands have about 150 mg of sodium in a 2-tablespoon serving. Discovering the products of some of the smaller manufacturers can be rewarding, with less than 100 mg of sodium in the same serving.

1. Place a large skillet over medium heat and spray lightly with oil. Add the onion and cook, stirring frequently, until the onion begins to soften. Add the chicken, chili powder, cayenne, and salt. Stir until the outside of the chicken is cooked.

2. Add ¼ cup of water and continue cooking for 7 to 10 minutes over medium heat, until the chicken is cooked through. Remove from the heat, let cool, and then refrigerate.

[CONTINUES]

NUTRITION FACTS

Serving size salad with 4
  ounces chicken
Servings 2
Calories 530
Calories from Fat 138
Total Fat 16 g (24%)
Saturated Fat 7 g (33%)
Trans Fat 0 g
Monounsaturated Fat 4 g
Cholesterol 91 mg (30%)
Sodium 414 mg (17%)
Total Carbohydrates 53 g (18%)
Dietary Fiber 10 g (41%)
Sugars 11 g
Protein 47 g
Vitamin A (44%)
Vitamin C (52%)
Calcium (38%)
Iron (27%)

*Parenthetical percentages
refer to % Daily Value.

3. When ready to assemble, place the tortilla chips in the bottom of a large bowl. Top with the lettuce and then the black beans. Arrange the tomato wedges around the edges. Top with the cooled chicken and sprinkle with the pumpkin seeds, green onion, and shredded cheese. Spoon the sour cream and salsa on top and serve.

Tomatillo Salsa

SERVINGS: 8 ▌ **SERVING SIZE:** 2 TABLESPOONS ▌ MAKES ABOUT 1 CUP ▌
THIS RECIPE CAN EASILY BE DOUBLED OR TRIPLED ▌ **COOKING TIME:** 15 MINUTES ▌
THIS KEEPS WELL FOR UP TO 2 WEEKS IN THE REFRIGERATOR

8 ounces tomatillos,
  chopped finely
1 medium-size tomato,
  chopped finely
1 small shallot, minced
¼ cup seeded and diced
  red bell pepper
¼ cup seeded and diced
  green bell pepper
½ teaspoon chili powder
½ teaspoon cayenne
1 medium-size jalapeño,
  minced
1 teaspoon honey
⅛ teaspoon salt
Juice of 1 lime

NUTRITION FACTS

Serving size 2 tablespoons
Servings 8
Calories 21
Calories from Fat 3
Total Fat 0 g (1%)
Saturated Fat 0 g (0%)
Trans Fat 0 g
Monounsaturated Fat 0 g
Cholesterol 0 mg (0%)
Sodium 41 mg (2%)
Total Carbohydrates 5 g (2%)
Dietary Fiber 1 g (4%)
Sugars 3 g
Protein 1 g
Vitamin A (9%)
Vitamin C (34%)
Calcium (1%)
Iron (2%)

*Parenthetical percentages
refer to % Daily Value.

Salsa has almost nothing in it except for healthy antioxidants. Eat all you want.

Blend all ingredients and let stand for at least 4 hours. Overnight is best.

Day 16 Alternative Dinner Choices

CONVENIENCE MEALS

Lean Cuisine Linguine Carbonara

RESTAURANT MEALS

P. F. Chang's Steamed Buddha's Feast with Vegetarian Lettuce Wraps

DAY 17 | LOOK AT SODIUM ON FOOD LABELS

The government created rules back in the 1980s for nutrition information labeling on packaged foods. Before the regulations were passed, the only information required was a listing of the ingredients in the package, in order from the largest amount to the smallest amount. Other than that, we were pretty much on our own and had to guess how much of something might or might not be in any particular food. Fortunately, it's a bit easier now.

Even so, reading a food label can be a bit of a challenge because of all the different numbers one is faced with. For sodium, the percentages listed on packages are based on a total daily intake of 2,400 milligrams (mg). This is a much lower sodium intake than most of us are eating today, with the average American consuming close to 6,000 mg per day. Some estimates place that intake much higher—in the 10,000 mg per day range for Western diets (that's ten *grams* of sodium).

While the percentage values are helpful, it's best to use them only as a guideline. The truly important numbers are those that show the amount of sodium in milligrams.

Even though we have much better research on this now, it turns out that the government's recommended guideline of 2,400 mg was a pretty good target. For those simply trying to eat healthier, the American Heart Association recommends no more than 2,300 mg per day (this is about the amount in a teaspoon of salt). Most physicians ask their patients with conditions such as congestive heart failure and more severe hypertension to eat less, however, with a target of 1,500 mg. I have found with informal testing of recipes that a sodium level of not less than 300 mg per serving for a main course dish is about the level that most people find "salty enough." I target my main course recipes at around 500 mg of sodium per serving.

The best way to approach this is to divide your day into sodium targets for each meal, with breakfast and lunch targets under 500 mg sodium and dinner under 1,000 mg. Look at the Nutrition Facts on any package of food and add the total milligrams of sodium per serving for the foods that you are eating.

Dr. Tim Says . . . Eat Low Sodium Soy Sauce

Soy sauce is one of the world's oldest condiments and is made by fermenting soybeans with roasted wheat (and sometimes barley). It is likely that its origins are as a preservative, and as with many preservatives, it is very high in salt. Soy sauce is a brewed product and has a savory flavor that activates the umami taste buds.

Used sparingly, soy sauce is a fantastic flavor enhancer. It can add a lot of flavor, but it can also add a ton of salt—enough that people who are salt sensitive or on restricted sodium diets can get into trouble. Traditional soy sauce has about 1,100 mg of sodium per tablespoon (give or take 100 milligrams). That's the equivalent of ½ teaspoon of salt.

Fortunately, there are excellent lower-sodium soy sauces on the market, with no difference in flavor between them and traditional soy sauce. The low-salt versions, however, have half the salt (only about 550 mg per tablespoon).

Pizza with Thai Peanut Sauce and Scallops

SERVINGS: 2 INDIVIDUAL PIZZAS ▌ **SERVING SIZE:** 1 PIZZA ▌ THIS RECIPE CAN EASILY BE MULTIPLIED ▌ **COOKING TIME:** 30 MINUTES ▌ **PREP TIME:** 60 MINUTES

2 teaspoons extra-virgin olive oil
1 large leek, cleaned and sliced into thin rounds
2 tablespoons Thai Peanut Sauce (recipe follows)
6 sea scallops (about 6 ounces)
½ recipe Whole Wheat Pizza Dough (page 55)*
2 tablespoons unsalted dry-roasted peanuts, chopped finely
½ cup fresh cilantro leaves
½ cup fresh mung bean sprouts
*The leftover half-recipe of whole wheat dough may be tightly wrapped and frozen and will keep for about 2 weeks.

NUTRITION FACTS

Serving size 1 pizza (including dough)
Servings 2
Calories 465
Calories from Fat 71
Total Fat 9 g (13%)
Saturated Fat 2 g (7%)
Trans Fat 0 g
Monounsaturated Fat 3 g
Cholesterol 28 mg (9%)
Sodium 480 mg (20%)
Total Carbohydrates 74 g (25%)
Dietary Fiber 10 g (40%)
Sugars 9 g
Protein 29 g
Vitamin A (21%)
Vitamin C (18%)
Calcium (8%)
Iron (28%)

*Parenthetical percentages refer to % Daily Value.

Serve with red wine (but not at breakfast) and a good movie. Leftovers are good cold for breakfast.

You don't have to make this pizza with the Thai Peanut Sauce recipe. There are a number of good, premade peanut sauces on the market that are not too high in calories, fat, or sodium. I will often substitute the Whole Foods 365 brand when I make this pizza and it still comes in at about the same nutrition content. If you are preparing the sauce yourself, it should be made first (see page 114).

This recipe also requires that the Whole Wheat Pizza Dough be made first (see page 55).

1. Pizza is best baked on a pizza stone, but a cookie sheet will work almost as well. Place in an oven that has been preheated to 500°F. Allow the baking surface to heat for at least 15 to 20 minutes.

2. Place 1 teaspoon of the olive oil in a nonstick skillet over medium-high heat. Add the leek and lower the heat to medium. Cook until the leek begins to soften and brown, stirring frequently.

3. Add the peanut sauce and toss to coat thoroughly. Set aside.

4. While the leek is cooking, heat the remaining teaspoon of olive oil in a small nonstick skillet over high heat. When the pan is very hot, add the scallops to the pan. Sear on one side for about 3 minutes and turn. Cook on the other side for about another 3 minutes. Transfer to a paper towel to drain. [CONTINUES]

5. When the scallops are cool, slice them in half into two disks per scallop (a total of six disks per pizza).

6. Gently stretch the pizza dough into two 8-inch rounds. Don't work too hard to get a perfectly round shape.

7. Make sure all the toppings are placed conveniently near the oven so that they will be easy to place on top of the dough.

8. Once the dough is formed, place the rounds on top of the hot pizza stone and top each with half of the leek mixture. Sprinkle with 1 tablespoon of peanuts per pizza, top with six scallop disks (seared side up), and then sprinkle ¼ cup of cilantro leaves over each pizza.

9. Bake for 10 to 12 minutes, until the dough begins to brown. Top with ¼ cup of bean sprouts and bake for another 2 minutes.

Thai Peanut Sauce

SERVINGS: 8 ▌ **SERVING SIZE: 2 TABLESPOONS PEANUT SAUCE** ▌ THIS RECIPE CAN EASILY BE MULTIPLIED ▌ **COOKING TIME: 30 MINUTES** ▌ THIS CAN BE MADE UP TO 48 HOURS IN ADVANCE AND REFRIGERATED

¼ cup peanut butter
6 tablespoons chicken stock
¼ cup reduced-fat (light) unsweetened coconut milk
2 teaspoons low-sodium soy sauce
2 teaspoons rice vinegar
2 teaspoons Tabasco sauce

NUTRITION FACTS

Serving size 2 tablespoons
Servings 8
Calories 45
Calories from Fat 25
Total Fat 3 g (4%)
Saturated Fat 1 g (4%)
Trans Fat 0 g
Monounsaturated Fat 0 g
Cholesterol 0 mg (0%)
Sodium 93 mg (4%)
Total Carbohydrates 3 g (1%)
Dietary Fiber 0 g (2%)
Sugars 1 g
Protein 2 g
Vitamin A (0%)
Vitamin C (0%)
Calcium (0%)
Iron (1%)

*Parenthetical percentages refer to % Daily Value.

This sauce will keep for about 3 weeks sealed tightly in the refrigerator.

Combine the peanut butter, chicken stock, coconut milk, soy sauce, vinegar, and Tabasco in a small bowl. Whisk until smooth and refrigerate.

Day 17 Alternative Dinner Choices

CONVENIENCE MEALS

Wolfgang Puck's Grilled Vegetable Cheeseless Pizza

RESTAURANT MEALS

Pizza Hut Half-Serving Cheese Only Personal Pan Pizza

DAY 18 | *CHOLESTEROL IS OKAY!*

At almost every talk I give, cholesterol comes up in the discussion. Back in the 1970s and '80s, there was a feeling that consuming dietary cholesterol was *the* cause of heart disease. People were told to not consume any more than 300 milligrams of cholesterol per day. The bad rap it took was not for very substantial reasons, however. Much of what happened in the late 1960s that laid the groundwork for cholesterol getting such a bad reputation wasn't based on sound science. Over the last thirty years, research has shown that for most people cholesterol is not a problem. The truth is, the amount of trans fat and saturated fat in your diet has much more impact on your blood cholesterol levels—and therefore your risk of heart disease— than does the amount of cholesterol you eat.

We do know that there are folks who are considered "hyper-responders" to cholesterol consumption, meaning they have a greater increase in their blood cholesterol after consuming dietary cholesterol (although this is not a tremendous increase). About a third of us might be more sensitive in this way.[4]

Keep in mind that there is a difference between *dietary cholesterol,* meaning the cholesterol that you consume, and the *blood* (or *serum*) *cholesterol* profile that your doctor gets back when she sends your blood to the lab.

For the most part, we don't know the exact mechanisms for lowering cholesterol. Fiber is one nutrient that does help lower cholesterol, and it appears that the mechanism has to do with fiber's effect on the absorption of dietary cholesterol and other fats. You likely already know that foods that are high in fiber, especially those with soluble fiber such as beans, oat bran, oatmeal, and rye, are clearly shown to improve cholesterol profiles. That's not to say that insoluble fiber, found in fruits, whole-grain products such as whole wheat flour, whole-grain breads and pastas, as well as in cereal grains such as rice, wild rice, and seeds, should be ignored. These guys are great, too!

We know that good-quality oils and fats that are high in monounsaturated fats can improve cholesterol profiles, but there's more to it than the fat itself. In the case of olive oil, many of its flavonoids, polyphenols, and other antioxidants are what appear to affect cholesterol. These are similar to compounds in such things as chocolate, red wine, and fruits that help change the composition of the lipids in the body.

Most of the large studies that are looking at cholesterol consumption look at eggs, as they are both a common food and high in cholesterol at about 250 mg per serving. Except for those who are diabetic, for most people it doesn't seem to matter all that much how much cholesterol is consumed.

The truth is, as far back as 1999, there was strong evidence that eggs were not an issue. Dr. Frank Hu and his colleagues looked at the combined data from two very large studies with over 37,000 participants.[5] Of the 2,626 reported cases of heart disease and stroke, the researchers found *no evidence* of a link between egg consumption and cardiovascular disease. Their conclusion stated, "These findings suggest that consumption of up to 1 egg per day is unlikely to have substantial overall impact on the risk of CHD or stroke among healthy men and women." When they looked at diabetics, however, there was some suggestion that diabetics who consume eggs might be at a higher risk.

There are also reports providing evidence that having eggs as part of a calorie-restricted diet resulted in improved weight loss (both regular and low-carb diets). These are small studies but appear effective.[6]

A recent study addressed eggs and heart disease, along with high blood pressure and congestive heart failure.[7] Researchers separated participants' egg consumption into six levels: less than one per week, one per week, two to four per week, five to six per week, one daily, and two or more per day. Those levels of egg consumption were correlated with that of the subjects who experienced heart failure, heart attacks, or high blood pressure.

They found that after controlling for a number of variables, including body mass index, physical activity, and smoking, those subjects eating fewer than six eggs per week saw no increase in their risk of heart failure. On the other hand, those who ate an egg every day had a 28 percent increase in their risk of heart failure, and those who ate two or more eggs per day increased their risk by 64 percent.

Further, when the researchers looked at the smaller group of subjects who provided cholesterol levels, they found no association between the amount of eggs the subjects ate and their total cholesterol, HDL cholesterol, or ratio of total cholesterol to HDL cholesterol.

I think that eggs are pretty good for you and that consuming high-cholesterol foods, such as eggs, liver, shrimp, and lobster, is not a problem for most folks. As the old saying goes, too much of a good thing is too much of a good thing. I don't think that this means you should eat eggs every day, but at the same time they appear unlikely to do you much harm in moderation (as with most foods). Better to look at the amount of fat and saturated fats in your overall diet than to obsess over how many eggs you eat.

Relax and enjoy your eggs!

Understanding Your Cholesterol Levels

Cholesterol is a waxy, yellow fat that is found in every cell in your body. It doesn't just float around in the blood by itself, it is carried around by lipoproteins. There are two main types: HDL (high-density lipoproteins) and LDL (low-density lipoproteins).

LDL CHOLESTEROL: LOW-DENSITY LIPOPROTEIN

LDL is considered to be "bad cholesterol" and is made up of particles of fats that carry cholesterol out to the body's tissues. When there is too much LDL cholesterol in the bloodstream, it can become a part of a thick, hard layer, called *plaques*, on the inside of your arteries. The buildup of plaques is known as *atherosclerosis*. The thicker the layer is, the more narrowed the arteries become.

When the arteries in the heart narrow because of plaque buildup, there is a decrease in blood flow. The blood carries oxygen; less blood flow means less oxygen carried to the tissues of the body. If the blood flow in the arteries in the heart gets blocked completely, the lack of oxygen causes a heart attack. The same can happen with the arteries that feed blood to the brain: if they become blocked, the lack of oxygen to the brain causes a stroke.

Keeping the LDL cholesterol level as low as possible is key to preventing heart attack and stroke. The optimal level depends on your other risk factors. See the table on page 119 for recommended levels of the different lipids.

HDL CHOLESTEROL: HIGH-DENSITY LIPOPROTEIN

HDL is also known as the "good cholesterol" because having higher levels of HDL protects against heart attack and stroke. Researchers believe that particles of fat that make up HDL carry cholesterol (both the source of the HDL, as well as LDL cholesterol that the particles touch) away from the arteries and back to the liver, where it can be removed from the body. This leaves less cholesterol at the site of the artery to form plaques. You want your HDL levels to be as high as possible.

TRIGLYCERIDES

Triglycerides are another important lipid. Like cholesterol, it is found in foods you eat, but your body also makes its own triglycerides. People with high triglycerides often have a high total cholesterol, a high LDL cholesterol, and a low HDL cholesterol level. Like a high total cholesterol and a high LDL cholesterol, high triglycerides is a risk factor for the buildup of plaques and the development of heart disease. People who have diabetes and those who are obese are more likely to have high triglycerides.

WHAT SHOULD YOUR RESULTS BE?

The following table is based on the current recommendations for the different types of cholesterol. High risk would be having three or more risk factors. It is best for people with two risk factors to be in the optimum range, and for lower-risk people to work to have their cholesterol in the desirable range.

CHOLESTERAL CHART

	TOTAL	LDL (BAD)	HDL (GOOD)	TRIGLYCERIDES
If your risk is very high (3 or more risk factors)	Under 160	As low as possible	Above 40	Under 150
Optimum	161–179	Under 100	Above 40	Under 150
Desirable levels	180–199	100–129	Above 40	150–199
Borderline high cholesterol	200–239	130–159		Over 200
High cholesterol	Over 240	160–189		Over 200
Very high cholesterol	Over 240	Over 190		Over 200

Risk factors for heart disease include:

- Family history (mother, father, sister, or brother with heart disease)
- Smoking (any smoking at all counts!)
- High blood pressure (hypertension)
- Diabetes
- Being male (or being a postmenopausal female)

HOW DO YOU COMPARE?

Fill your cholesterol results in to the spaces below. Keep track of your progress toward optimum over time.

DATE	TOTAL	LDL (BAD)	HDL (GOOD)	TRIGLYCERIDES

DAY 18 | DINNER

WHITE BEAN CHILI AND SALAD WITH THOUSAND ISLAND DRESSING

White Bean Chili

SERVINGS: 8 ▮ **SERVING SIZE:** ABOUT 2 CUPS ▮ THIS RECIPE CAN EASILY BE DOUBLED, BUT YOU'LL NEED A LARGE POT ▮ LEFTOVERS ARE GREAT! SAVE THE LEFTOVERS FOR DINNER ON DAY 20. ▮ **COOKING TIME:** 2 HOURS ▮ **PREP TIME:** 30 MINUTES

1 pound dried white northern beans, or 3 (15-ounce) cans no-salt-added white beans, drained and rinsed
1 tablespoon canola oil
1½ cups white onion, chopped
2 cloves garlic, minced
3 large russet potatoes, peeled and cubed
2 cups chicken stock
1½ cups white wine
1 pound boneless, skinless chicken breasts, cubed
2 teaspoons chili powder
1 teaspoon Tabasco sauce
2 teaspoons ground cumin
1 cup 1% milk
4 ounces reduced-fat white Cheddar cheese, grated
2 teaspoons (per serving) nonfat sour cream, for garnish
2 teaspoons (per serving) reduced-fat white Cheddar cheese, grated, for garnish
2 teaspoons (per serving) chopped chives, for garnish

This is one of my favorite chilis. First off, it's a great variation on red bean and meat chili. Also, by using the chicken, there's about one-third the fat. It's the perfect recipe to make on a weekend so that you'll have plenty left over for lunches throughout the week.

1. If using dried beans, place the beans in a bowl and cover with quarts of cold water. Soak overnight.

2. Place the oil in a large stockpot over medium heat. Add the onion and garlic and cook slowly. Stir frequently and don't let the onion brown.

3. Add the beans, potatoes, 1 cup of the chicken stock, and 1 cup of the white wine. Over medium-low heat, let simmer for 30 minutes.

4. Add the cubed chicken, chili powder, Tabasco, and cumin. Stir well and add the rest of the chicken stock and white wine. Cook over low heat until the beans are soft (about 1 hour).

5. Add the milk and 4 ounces of grated cheese, stir, and heat through. Do not allow the chili to boil.

6. Top each serving with 2 teaspoons each sour cream, Cheddar, and chives.

Chef Tim Says . . .
How to Cook with Dried vs. Canned Beans

Purchasing dried beans and soaking them overnight is the best way to get the true bean flavor and a smooth texture (not always convenient, mind you, so don't hesitate to use canned beans that have been drained and rinsed). Generally speaking, a 15-ounce can of beans yields 1½ cups.

After soaking the dried beans, rinse them well and then cook with enough water to cover the beans (at least an inch or more above the beans). Depending on the type of bean, it will take about 30 to 40 minutes of cooking over medium-low heat. In a pinch, rinsing the dried beans and cooking them without presoaking will be almost as good. They won't have as true a bean flavor, and the cooking time will be about 25 percent longer.

You do have to be careful when using canned beans, because of their sodium content. There are usually 400 to 500 mg of sodium in ½ cup of canned beans. Unfortunately, simply rinsing canned beans doesn't help to reduce the sodium content. However, if the beans are rinsed and then heated in water, the sodium content drops by about a third.

In the recipes in this book that call for canned beans, the Nutrition Facts are based on no-salt-added canned beans. If you need to be on a very low-salt diet, buying dried beans and cooking them yourself lets you control the amount of sodium even more.

Day 18 Alternative Dinner Choices

CONVENIENCE MEALS

Kashi Southwest Style Chicken

RESTAURANT MEALS

Ruby Tuesday White Bean Chicken Chili with Side Salad

I have told you that I like to use butter in recipes. It enhances the flavor and texture of recipes in a way that few other ingredients can. Most of the time you don't need much; just a bit works wonders. A chef friend once said that he believed it was easy for chefs to hide their sins by simply adding more fat and salt to a recipe. He would say, "You can make bad food taste better with more butter or salt, but it's better to just make great food with the right amount of ingredients." I believe that he's right and that measuring is essential to great food.

So when I cook, I measure. This is also one of the simplest tips for reducing calories and eating healthy.

Butter is a good example, but all fats have a lot of calories. The rule of thumb is that a teaspoon of oil or butter contains about 45 calories and 5 grams of fat. Sometimes it's a fat that is better for you, but it's still fat and still calories. Television chefs randomly pour oil into pans without thinking about the added calories. That extra oil doesn't add much to the flavor or texture of their recipes, however, and this is not a practice you should adopt. Measure that oil before you pour it!

Salt is the ingredient that I am the most careful with. It's really easy to add more sodium to a dish than you need and most recipes are much too salty to begin with. It's easy to cut back on your sodium intake by measuring carefully. A teaspoon of salt has about 2,300 milligrams of sodium (the recommended total per day). One-eighth teaspoon of salt per portion makes most dishes just salty enough: This is about 300 mg of added sodium. When I am creating recipes, I use this as my starting point, then I reduce or add salt depending on whether the recipe has other ingredients that contain sodium, such as Parmesan cheese or soy sauce.

I like using my salt grinder. I have measured it and know that my salt mill dispenses ⅛ teaspoon with ten cranks of the grinder, so that's ¹⁄₁₆ teaspoon with five turns. You'll need to experiment a bit with your own grinder to know just how much yours puts out, but it's great for salting fish or meat before cooking. (The same applies to my pepper mill. Freshly ground pepper is a tremendous improvement over the flat flavor of the pre-ground kind.)

Baking is an exacting science that requires careful measurement to make sure that everything turns out right. This is true with cooking as well, and I use measuring cups and spoons for all ingredients, including milk, chicken stock, flour, rice, oatmeal, and the like. Research shows that rounding the top of a measuring cup instead of leveling it off can add up to 30 percent more calories. Measuring keeps excess calories from creeping into your diet.

Professional bakers use scales to weigh their ingredients and this is a lesson we can learn from them. If you are going to purchase only one piece of equipment for your kitchen, make it a scale. Weigh your chicken, beef, potatoes, pasta, and so forth. Recipes are written using measuring cups and spoons, but learning to weigh foods helps you to understand what a proper portion size is. You'll quickly get a feel for just how much 4 ounces of chicken or fish is. This will not only keep you on track with your calories at home, but you will come to realize just how many extra calories there is in restaurant food because you'll know what a normal portion size is.

Grouper with White Beans and Tomato Vinaigrette

SERVINGS: 2 ▌ **SERVING SIZE:** 4 OUNCES FISH WITH BEANS ▌ THIS RECIPE CAN EASILY BE MULTIPLIED ▌ **COOKING TIME:** 45 MINUTES

1 ounce dried wild mushrooms (e.g., porcini)

12 grape tomatoes, quartered

1 tablespoon + 1 teaspoon olive oil

1 tablespoon flat-leaf parsley, chopped coarsely

1 teaspoon balsamic vinegar

1 (1 ounce) slice prosciutto ham, diced

½ cup small-diced carrot

½ cup small-diced celery

½ cup small-diced leek, well washed (white part only)

1 (15-ounce) can white beans, drained and rinsed

¼ teaspoon salt

Freshly ground black pepper

¼ teaspoon dried oregano

Spray olive oil

2 (4-ounce) grouper fillets (or other fatty whitefish, such as halibut)

This is the Mediterranean diet at its best: low-fat white fish, olive oil, veggies, and healthy beans with tons of fiber. This recipe calls for dried oregano, but you can use about a teaspoon of fresh or about the same amount of rosemary. In the dead of winter, the bright tomatoes in vinaigrette taste just like spring is coming.

1. Place 1½ cups of water in a saucepan over high heat. When the water boils, add the dried mushrooms and lower the heat until the water is simmering. After the stock has cooked for about 15 minutes, remove the pan from the heat.

2. Place the tomatoes, 1 tablespoon of olive oil, parsley, and vinegar in a small bowl and toss well. Place in the refrigerator to chill.

3. Preheat the oven to 400°F. Place a large ovenproof skillet inside while the oven is preheating.

4. Place the 1 teaspoon of olive oil in a medium-size skillet over medium heat. Add the prosciutto and cook, stirring frequently, for about 1 minute. Add the carrot and celery and cook, stirring frequently, for about 2 minutes. Add the leek and cook for another minute, stirring frequently.

5. Add the white beans, salt, pepper to taste, and oregano. Strain the mushroom broth into the skillet with the white beans (save the porcini mushrooms in the fridge for your scrambled eggs). Lower the heat to a simmer. Stir occasionally.

6. Lightly spray the skillet in the oven with olive oil. Add the fish, skin side down, and return to the oven. Cook for about 6 minutes, then turn the fish over.

7. While the fish is cooking, divide the bean mixture between two plates. When the fish is done (about 5 minutes on the second side), place the fillets on top of the beans. Top the fish with the chilled tomato vinaigrette and serve.

Day 19 Alternative Dinner Choices

CONVENIENCE MEALS

Michael Angelo's Italian Natural Cuisine Vegetable Lasagna

RESTAURANT MEALS

Red Lobster Grilled Halibut or
Red Lobster Garlic-Grilled Jumbo Shrimp

DAY 20 | *PORTION-SIZE YOURSELF*

In the last few decades, portion size has become a major issue, with portions in restaurants increasing dramatically. Forty years ago, a 32-ounce milk shake with 1,160 calories would have been unusual. There was no such thing as a Quarter Pounder (let alone a Double Quarter Pounder), and getting a mountain of nachos would have been rare. These huge plates that are currently served have spilled over into how people choose to portion their food at home.

For example, one study, done in the late 1980s and repeated in 2006,[8] evaluated the difference in the last two decades in how college students choose meals at a buffet. One hundred and seventy-seven students freely served themselves meals, which were then weighed. The portions were scored against the recommended portion sizes. The portion sizes chosen for breakfast and lunch in 2006 were found to be more than 125 percent of the standard portion. Overall, all the portions the students chose were larger than in the 1984 research.

Much of the difficulty people seem to have is with larger portions as opposed to normal or smaller servings. People just can't tell the difference between normal and too big. Brian Wansink, a food researcher, and his colleagues at Cornell University set up a study[9] where they approached people in fast-food restaurants and asked them to estimate the number of calories in the meal that they had just eaten. The researchers had been watching and recording what the participants had eaten.

People underestimated the number of calories they'd eaten by an average of 23 percent. When the researchers looked at the estimates given for supersized meals vs. regular ones, they found that those eating a smaller meal were better able to accurately estimate the amount of calories they had eaten. This wasn't the case with larger meals, where diners underestimated the calories they had just eaten by 38 percent. Dr. Wansink has been able to re-create these real-world findings in his lab in numerous experiments.

So what works? Portion control. In 2004, researchers at the CDC in Atlanta surveyed 2,124 adults who had tried to lose weight in the prior year.[10] Of these, 587 had lost weight and kept it off. Leading the five most common weight-loss strategies was smaller portions, while other strategies included reducing the amount of food eaten overall, more fruits and vegetables, fewer fatty foods, and no sweetened beverages.

Taking the time to learn the right portion size is an important tool in managing your weight. Having a scale as well as measuring cups and spoons on hand is critical to learning correct portion sizes. Here's a guide to the right portion sizes for your recipes:

The natural extension of this is the size of your plate. A lot of research has gone into the question, Does it make a difference whether you use a small or a large plate in how much you actually eat? The answer is yes, for adults, although not so much for kids.

Many studies of kids have shown mixed results on whether plate size is a factor when children serve themselves. For instance, in one study, it

PORTION SIZE

INGREDIENT	BEFORE COOKING	AFTER COOKING	LOOKS LIKE
GRAINS			
Rice	¼ cup	½ cup	½ baseball
Pasta	2 ounces	½–⅔ cup	½ baseball
Dry cereal	1 cup		The size of a fist
Potato	4 ounces		Computer mouse
Potato (mashed)	4 ounces	½ cup	½ baseball
Bread	1 slice		
Pancake	½ cup batter	Two	Compact disc
Bagel	2 ounces		Hockey puck
MEATS			
Beef	4 ounces		Deck of cards
Pork	4 ounces		Deck of cards
Veal	4 ounces		Deck of cards
Fish	4 ounces		Checkbook
Poultry	4 ounces		Deck of cards
Peanut butter	2 tablespoons		Ping-Pong ball
FRUITS AND VEGGIES			
Salad greens	1 cup		Baseball
Berries	½ cup		
Apple	1 medium		Baseball
Orange	1 medium		Baseball
Raisins	½ cup		Large egg
DAIRY			
Cheese	1½ ounces		Four stacked dice
Milk	1 cup		(choose low-fat)
Yogurt	1 cup		(choose low-fat)
FATS			
Oils	1 teaspoon		Thumb tip
Butter	1 teaspoon		Thumb tip

didn't matter how big the plate was or if they served themselves by filling plates from a buffet; they pretty much ate the same amount of food.[11]

For adults, it makes a difference. Possibly our perceptions become more accurate as we get older. Brian Wansink studied adult nutritionists at a staged ice-cream social.[12] The participants were randomly given a large bowl or a small bowl to use for their ice cream. They were then given a large or a small serving spoon to serve themselves. Afterward, they were questioned about how much ice cream they felt they had served themselves and how much they had eaten.

Those given a larger bowl served themselves about one-third more ice cream. When they used the larger serving spoon, they took about 15 percent more ice cream. By using both a larger bowl and spoon, folks served themselves a whopping 45 percent more than did those using the combination of a smaller bowl and smaller serving spoon. Interestingly, only three of those at the party didn't finish their ice cream (and these were nutritionists who should presumably know better).

Having a guide to portion size on the correct-size plate has been shown to help as well. "The Diet Plate" is an 11-inch dinner plate, with outlines of the appropriate portion sizes printed directly on the plate.[13]

Researchers used a similar cereal bowl with rings painted on the inside to show serving sizes for specific kinds of cereal. In a study of obese diabetics, the scientists randomized half to use the Diet Plate and bowls. The rest simply followed their usual routine and recommendations from their doctors and dietitians. Over six months of use, the group who used the Diet Plate lost significantly more weight. Not a little bit, either, but the equivalent to a 300-pound man's losing up to 17.1 pounds.

If using a smaller plate for meals helps you eat the right portion sizes, I am all for it.

DAY 20 | DINNER

LEFTOVER WHITE BEAN CHILI (PAGE 120) AND PARMESAN SQUASH

Parmesan Squash

SERVINGS: 2 ▌ SERVING SIZE: 1 LARGE SQUASH ▌ THIS RECIPE CAN EASILY BE DOUBLED
OR TRIPLED ▌ COOKING TIME: 25 MINUTES

2 (8-ounce) yellow summer squash
Freshly ground black pepper
2 tablespoons fresh herbs of your choice, minced
1 ounce Parmigiano-Reggiano, grated

These are two perfect ingredients that make a wonderful dish. The yellow squash tastes like summer and its own buttery flavor is enhanced by the Parmesan. I especially like using just a little bit of rosemary for the herb. Plus, squash is really low in calories and high in fiber and vitamin C.

NUTRITION FACTS

Serving size 1 large squash
Servings 2
Calories 99
Calories from Fat 37
Total Fat 4 g (7%)
Saturated Fat 2 g (112%)
Trans Fat 0 g
Monounsaturated Fat 1 g
Cholesterol 10 mg (3%)
Sodium 233 mg (10%)
Total Carbohydrates 10 g (3%)
Dietary Fiber 4 g (17%)
Sugars 0 g
Protein 7 g
Vitamin A (8%)
Vitamin C (32%)
Calcium (22%)

*Parenthetical percentages refer to % Daily Value.

1. Place 2 cups of water in a medium-size pot fitted with a steamer basket and heat over high heat. Preheat the oven to 325°F.

2. Cut and discard about ¼ inch from the stem end of each squash and then slice lengthwise. Place the four halves in the steamer and steam until slightly tender.

3. Remove the steamed squash and place in a shallow baking dish. Place the dish in the oven and bake for about 10 minutes. Remove from the oven and sprinkle with pepper to taste, the herbs, and the cheese.

4. Return the pan to the oven and cook until the cheese is melted (about 5 minutes).

Dr. Tim Says . . .

Myth: Eating late at night or just before you go to bed makes you gain weight.

Truth: Calories are calories. Period. If you eat too many and don't exercise enough, you will gain weight. Eating late or just before going to bed simply doesn't matter.

When you eat too much, your body has an amazing ability to store the extra calories as fat. Eating later, for most people, generally means that they postpone their meal and then in response to their hunger, eat more calories than they need.

CONVENIENCE MEALS

Kashi Southwest Style Chicken

RESTAURANT MEALS

Ruby Tuesday White Bean Chicken Chili with Side Salad

DAY 21 | CLEAN OUT YOUR PANTRY

When I am giving talks, I always joke that none of my patients ever eats Oreo cookies. Now, I find this really strange, because the aisles in the grocery store are *full* of cookies (but *my* patients say they never buy them). This always gets a big laugh, but I'm sure folks are laughing at themselves. We aren't always honest with ourselves, and probably even more often are not completely honest with our doctors (shocking, I know).

When my patients tell me they don't eat cookies, I would really like to leave the office and drive to their house and go through their cupboards and refrigerator with them. Some patients might prove me wrong, but the research says that most people have an awful lot of cookies or other junk in their pantry. When researchers have studied people's trash, they have seen a clear disconnect between what people will claim they are eating and what ends up in their trash bins.

So what should you do? Clean out your kitchen. Get rid of the stupid food. Start with the cupboard. If you have sugar-laden cereals, get rid of them (check the labels and use the 20/5 rule). Choose high-fiber cereals such as oatmeal, granola, and healthy whole-grain cereals.

Toss out your pre-prepared foods. Such convenience products as Hamburger Helper, Sloppy Joe mixes, and Rice-A-Roni are full of saturated fat and salt that you just don't need. There are better choices. Keep good-quality pasta sauces on hand along with whole wheat pasta, for a quick meal. You will have already purchased your own spices to make Sloppy

Joes and tacos, and the version you make at home will taste just as good—if not better—than those made with a mix. Fill your pantry with the ingredients that you need to make other fresh, healthy recipes: rice, beans, lentils, canned tomatoes, canned tuna, and low-sodium chicken broth.

The same rule holds true for snacks. If they're processed, such as crackers, potato chips, and corn chips, toss them out. If you are a salty/savory snacker, fill your pantry with nuts. The 100-calorie single serving of microwave popcorn is also a fantastic snack option, especially when you compare it with the same volume of potato chips at almost 400 calories.

This also holds true for those Oreo cookies. If you are a sweet snacker, get rid of the cookies, cakes, and candy and fill your kitchen with fruit. Canned, fresh, frozen, or dried; it doesn't matter. There's great evidence that you'll be just as satisfied (and happier) eating fruit rather than candy.

After finishing with your cupboard, it's time for the refrigerator. I'll talk later about more specific choices of meats and fish and such, but for now look at your freezer. Most commercially prepared frozen dinners are pretty bad for you. (The frozen meal "alternative choices" I include on each day have all been reviewed by the Dr. Gourmet Tasting Panel and are better for you, although many still contain more salt than you should eat on a regular basis.) On Day 31, I'll talk about what to fill your freezer with, so that between frozen items and those in your cupboard, you'll always have something quick and easy to make.

The best way to fill up your kitchen with healthy ingredients is planning. Following this six-week plan will help you slowly but surely buy the pasta, rice, beans, spices, herbs, vegetables, chicken stock, and so on that you need to make great-tasting healthy recipes.

DAY 21 | DINNER

PUMPKIN-CRUSTED TROUT WITH LEMON SAUCE, WILD RICE, AND ROASTED TOMATOES

Pumpkin-Crusted Trout with Lemon Sauce

SERVINGS: 2 ▌ **SERVING SIZE:** 4 OUNCES TROUT ▌ THIS RECIPE CAN EASILY BE MULTI-
PLIED ▌ **COOKING TIME:** 30 MINUTES

1 egg white
½ teaspoon grated lemon
  peel
¼ teaspoon salt
¼ teaspoon dried tarragon
⅛ teaspoon dry mustard
⅛ teaspoon freshly ground
  black pepper
2 ounces dried pumpkin
  seeds
2 teaspoons grapeseed oil
2 (4-ounce) trout fillets
Juice of ½ lemon

NUTRITION FACTS

Serving size 4 ounces trout
Servings 2
Calories 353
Calories from Fat 165
Total Fat 19 g (29%)
Saturated Fat 3 g (15%)
Monounsaturated Fat 7 g
Trans Fat 0 g
Cholesterol 66 mg (22%)
Sodium 554 mg (23%)
Total Carbohydrates 5 g (2%)
Dietary Fiber 1 g (3%)
Sugars 1 g
Protein 41 g
Vitamin A (2%)
Vitamin C (11%)
Calcium (7%)
Iron (22%)

*Parenthetical percentages
refer to % Daily Value.

This is a quick and simple dish that works for a weeknight meal as well as a perfect dinner party dish. There's great fish with pumpkin seeds and grapeseed oil, all high in monounsaturated fats. You can use any herb that takes your fancy. Oregano and lime juice are great examples of substitutions you can make.

You can use these techniques with other ingredient choices: pecans with salmon; almonds with halibut. Almost any combination of fish or chicken with nuts and the herb of your choice will work great.

1. Preheat the oven to 400°F. Place a large ovenproof skillet in the oven.

2. Whisk together the egg white, lemon peel, salt, tarragon, mustard, and black pepper.

3. Place the pumpkin seeds in a mini chopper and chop until the seeds are broken into small pieces. This should take only five to eight pulses. Alternatively, you can place the seeds in a zippered plastic bag and crush them with a rolling pin.

4. When the pan is hot, dredge the flesh side of the fish in the egg white mixture, then dredge in the pumpkin seeds. Coat only one side of the trout.

5. Place the grapeseed oil in the hot pan, swirling to coat the bottom of the skillet well. Place the trout, coated side down, in the pan. Cook for 8 minutes and add the lemon juice to the pan. Cook for 2 to 4 minutes more and serve.

Wild Rice

SERVINGS: 2 ▐ **SERVING SIZE:** ABOUT ½ CUP ▐ THIS RECIPE CAN EASILY BE DOUBLED OR TRIPLED ▐ **COOKING TIME:** 45 MINUTES

¼ teaspoon salt
½ cup wild rice

NUTRITION FACTS

Serving size ½ cup
Servings 2
Calories 143
Calories from Fat 0
Total Fat 0 g (0%)
Saturated Fat 0 g (0%)
Monounsaturated Fat 0 g
Cholesterol 0 mg (0%)
Sodium 293 mg (12%)
Total Carbohydrates 30 g (10%)
Dietary Fiber 2 g (8%)
Sugars 2 g
Protein 6 g
Vitamin A (0%)
Vitamin C (0%)
Calcium (1%)
Iron (4%)

*Parenthetical percentages refer to % Daily Value.

Wild rice (actually a kind of grass) is great for you, with 2 grams of fiber per serving, and it's easy to cook. Although it is more expensive than regular rice, it's worth treating yourself now and then. I think that it goes especially well with light fish dishes such as trout or catfish.

1. In a medium-size saucepan, heat 1½ cups of water and the salt. When the water boils, stir in the wild rice.

2. Lower the heat to medium-low and simmer, partially covered, for about 15 minutes. Do not boil away all of the liquid and do not stir the rice.

3. When a very small amount of liquid remains, remove the pan from the burner and let it stand, covered, for 5 minutes before serving.

Roasted Tomatoes

SERVINGS: 2 ▐ **SERVING SIZE:** 2 TOMATOES ▐ THIS RECIPE CAN EASILY BE MULTIPLIED BY 2, 3, OR 4 ▐ **COOKING TIME:** 30 MINUTES

Spray olive oil
4 medium-size tomatoes
⅛ teaspoon salt
Freshly ground black
    pepper

It is so simple really. Roast some tomatoes as a side dish. These are great tasting, low in calories, and take no time at all to make.

1. Preheat the oven to 375°F. Place a large ovenproof skillet in the oven.

2. When the oven is hot, lightly spray the pan with olive oil, sprinkle the tomatoes with the salt and pepper to taste, and place the tomatoes inside, stem side down. [CONTINUES]

3. Roast for 30 minutes and remove from the oven. Turn the tomatoes over so they are stem side up, resting in the hot pan, and let them cool in the pan for 5 minutes.

4. Serve.

Chef Tim Says . . . Eat Fresh Tomatoes

Buying tomatoes at the supermarket can be a daunting task. The quality is often poor because most are picked green and ripened in big rooms, using ethylene gas.

However, even the worst tomato can be made better by placing it stem side down on a sunny windowsill. It will continue to ripen further, and if you want it chilled, place it in the fridge for only a couple of hours.

Plum or Roma tomatoes: This is the slightly elongated tomato that is now in most markets. Growers like them because they travel better than larger tomatoes, but I find the texture is slightly mealy. There are few seeds and less juice. These are fair, all-purpose tomatoes for salads or cooking.

Cherry tomatoes: About an inch in diameter, these are available in both red and yellow. I like them because they often have a bright tomato flavor year-round and are seldom mealy. There are even smaller tomatoes as well: grape and currant tomatoes.

Heirloom tomatoes: These are grown from heirloom or antique seeds. Now available in larger quantities, they are usually superior because the strains are chosen for flavor and not hardiness. Most growers are also invested in creating a higher-quality product. You won't often find them in regular grocery stores but at gourmet markets, because they move directly from grower to market (and are not gassed as most other tomatoes are).

Day 21 Alternative Dinner Choices

Lean Cuisine Szechuan Style Stir Fry with Shrimp or
Lean Cuisine Lemon Pepper Fish

RESTAURANT MEALS

Red Lobster Garlic-Grilled Jumbo Shrimp or
Red Lobster Grilled Fish

CHAPTER 4 | *WEEK 4 GOALS*

This is my favorite week. You're halfway through the cooking plan and you're getting healthier. Losing 2 to 4 pounds in the first three weeks is typical and a great target for you. Over time, these diet principles will lead to better cholesterol scores, improved blood sugar, and lower blood pressure. The recipes you have been preparing may be familiar, and in the next ten days you'll see how ingredient choices can translate Mediterranean diet principles for American recipes.

It's time to begin building your new Mediterranean pantry. In the last three weeks, you have purchased ingredients that you'll need to make great recipes beyond this six-week program. After cleaning out your pantry yesterday, you'll start to learn about how to rebuild it with fresh products, including veggies, fruits, nuts, whole grains, and legumes. You'll learn the best choices for seafood and dairy products. What you're learning is not just *how* to make the change, but *why* it is so important to your health now and for the long term.

This week, you'll:

▌ Start building your new pantry

Vegetables	Fruits and nuts	Cereals and grains
Legumes	Fish	Dairy

■ Expand your recipe horizons. You'll continue with a lot of familiar favorites, including fried chicken and fish as well as beef
Stroganoff. There are also a few new concepts, including a great
barley salad—perfect for pot luck dinners—and a salmon salad
with chickpeas.

WEEK 4 | MENU

A personalized shopping list for Week 3 can be found at DrGourmet.com/
shoppinglist.

DAY 22 | GO MEDITERRANEAN

We've come to the end of three weeks, which to this point have focused
mostly on the fundamentals of nutrition as well as ways to plan and bring
some structure to your diet. We'll now shift emphasis to how to make
changes in what you eat as well as how to adapt them to your life. We know
that fad diets are pretty silly and don't work for the long term. So what
does work?

Over the last three decades, a lot has been written about how the
French eat a diet that is high in fat, yet they don't have the problems with
obesity that America has. This so-called French Paradox has led to a great
deal of research, and that research extends well beyond France to almost
every country surrounding the Mediterranean Sea.

The research is founded in the early work of Ancel Keys. He recognized the difference in health issues between Mediterranean and other
Western countries, and his early research has been the cornerstone of what
we now call the Mediterranean diet. While the name seems exotic, the style
of eating really isn't all that unusual and is actually pretty simple. It is easily
adaptable to our Western-style diet.

It is higher in vegetables, beans and peas (legumes), fruits, nuts, and
whole grains. People in Mediterranean countries use olive oil as their main

WEEK 4 MENU

RECIPE	CONVENIENCE FOOD ALTERNATIVE	RESTAURANT MEAL ALTERNATIVE
DAY 22		
Oven-Fried Chicken and Roasted Corn on the Cob with Pan-Grilled Broccoli	Michael Angelo's Signature Line Chicken Parmesan	Applebee's Tortilla Chicken Melt
DAY 23		
Eggplant Parmesan	Michael Angelo's Italian Natural Cuisine Vegetable Lasagna	Souplantation/Sweet Tomatoes Joan's Broccoli Madness
DAY 24		
Shrimp Fried Rice	Lean Cuisine Salmon with Basil	Red Lobster Garlic-Grilled Jumbo Shrimp
DAY 25		
Spring Barley Salad	Healthy Choice Tomato Basil Penne	Wendy's Broccoli and Cheese Potato
DAY 26		
Seared Salmon and Chickpea Salad	Lean Cuisine Lemon Pepper Fish	Souplantation/Sweet Tomatoes Tuna Tarragon
DAY 27		
Oven-Fried Fish with Yam Home Fries and Pan-Grilled Asparagus	Lean Cuisine Salmon with Basil	Ruby Tuesday Asian Glazed Salmon
DAY 28		
Beef Stroganoff with Egg Noodles	Michael Angelo's Italian Natural Cuisine Lasagna with Meat Sauce	Ruby Tuesday Petite Sirloin

source of fat and eat much less highly saturated fats, such as butter, shortening, and lard. Butter is actually used in small amounts, and very carefully, for maximum flavor and texture. These people eat more fish than beef and poultry (although they do eat both of the latter), and most of the dairy they consume is in the form of yogurts and cheeses.

Certainly the Mediterranean diet includes meat, but it is leaner and eaten far less often. Their alcohol consumption is also very moderate— usually drunk with meals, and usually wine.

One of the best pieces of research we have is a large study of healthy adults in Greece.[1] This was the first big study that showed that those following a Mediterranean-style diet were far less likely to die from cancer and heart disease. Before this study was done, we just didn't have any good guidelines for healthy ways to eat; people were told not to eat eggs or butter or meat, but we didn't really know what actually worked to *improve* one's health. The other bonus from this research is that it showed a link between this way of eating and cancer prevention, which until then just wasn't very conclusive.

The researchers followed the twenty-two thousand participants and looked at the nine dietary components that I mentioned above—veggies, legumes, fruits and nuts, whole grains, fats and oils, fish, dairy foods, meats, and alcohol.

The study was fairly simple. The researchers gave a value of either 1 or 0 for each of the nine diet categories. Whoever in the study ate more or less of a particular dietary component based on the mean amount consumed, received a 1 for that component. The perfect score for a Mediterranean diet would be 9, whereas a tally of 0 is more along the lines of a Western diet. The study found that those with higher scores lived longer.

The best part? It revealed that even small changes can have a huge effect on your health. A 2-point improvement—say, from 5 to 7—resulted in a 25 percent lower chance of death from heart disease. Just by making small changes in your diet, such as eating more fruit and whole grains, you can have a major impact on your health!

Other research has shown that those following a Mediterranean-style diet lower their blood pressure, control their cholesterol, and live longer.

We know also that the Mediterranean diet can help prevent heart disease. But what if you already have heart problems?

A team of researchers looked at six major hospitals in Greece for a term of one year.[2] Almost all the patients in those hospitals who were diagnosed with acute coronary syndrome (meaning either a heart attack or unstable angina) were included in the study. After the patients had been treated and were stable, they were interviewed regarding their lifestyle habits (smoking, exercise, etc.) and demographic information. Their diet was assessed using a very detailed food questionnaire that helped the researchers determine just how closely the patient's diet matched the Mediterranean diet. Points were assigned to the various components of the diet, with a maximum score of 55 most closely matching the Mediterranean diet. Patients were considered to have "high adherence" with a score of 36 or above, and "low adherence" with a score below 30. The patients were then monitored through the first thirty days after their hospitalization, and their outcome and final diagnosis were correlated with their Mediterranean diet score.

The results are pretty astounding. A Mediterranean diet score just 5 units higher than another patient's meant:

▌ A 15 percent lower risk of having a heart attack (remember that not all patients had been hospitalized for a heart attack)

▌ A 23 percent lower risk of dying during hospitalization

▌ A 19 percent lower likelihood of having another cardiac event during the first 30 days after hospitalization for an initial cardiac event

Interestingly, those whose diet matched the Mediterranean diet more closely tended to be those who were hospitalized for unstable angina, as opposed to those who were hospitalized for heart attack. It's clear that you don't have to follow the Mediterranean diet perfectly to see its advantages for your heart.

It takes very little to improve your Mediterranean diet score. To score a 1 in each category, for a woman eating a 1,500-calorie diet, this translates to the following:

MEDITERRANEAN DIET

	FOOD CATEGORY	AVERAGE PER DAY
1	Vegetables	More than 8.9 ounces
2	Legumes (peas, peanuts, beans)	More than 1.75 ounces
3	Fruits and nuts	More than 7.7 ounces
4	Dairy (cheese and yogurt)	Less than 6.9 ounces
5	Cereals (whole wheat, bran, oatmeal, brown rice, quinoa)	More than 8.9 ounces
6	Lean Meats	Less than 3.25 ounces
7	Fish (especially fatty fish such as tuna, salmon, halibut, mackerel, cod)	More than 0.75 ounces
8	Alcohol	Between one and two drinks per day
9	Fats	A ratio of 1.6 grams of unsaturated fat to every gram of saturated fat

In the coming days, I'll tell you about other research to support each of these nine areas and give you some practical ways to make these changes in your own diet.

DAY 22 | DINNER

OVEN-FRIED CHICKEN AND ROASTED CORN ON THE COB WITH PAN-GRILLED BROCCOLI

Chef Tim Says . . . Use Melba Toast for a Crispy Crust

Melba toast is amazing as breading! I keep a box on hand and generally use the plain melba toast, not the flavored, because I add my own spices.

Melba toast is said to have been created in 1897; allegedly the renowned chef Auguste Escoffier devised the recipe for the famous opera singer Dame Nellie Melba when she was ill (at the time, Escoffier was chef at the Ritz, where she lived). Peach Melba is also named for her.

Oven-Fried Chicken

SERVINGS: 4 ▌ **SERVING SIZE:** 1 CHICKEN PIECE ▌ THIS RECIPE CAN EASILY BE MULTI-PLIED ▌ **COOKING TIME:** 45 MINUTES ▌ LEFTOVERS KEEP WELL FOR 2 DAYS. ALLOW TO COOL BEFORE REFRIGERATING.

1 large egg
1 large egg white
1 tablespoon Dijon mustard
1 (5-ounce) box plain melba toast
1 teaspoon dried thyme
1 teaspoon dried rosemary
½ teaspoon dried oregano
¼ teaspoon garlic powder
¼ teaspoon salt
½ teaspoon freshly ground black pepper
¼ teaspoon cayenne
4 (4-ounce) boneless, skinless chicken breasts
Spray oil

NUTRITION FACTS

Serving size 1 chicken breast
Servings 4
Calories 293
Calories from Fat 36
Total Fat 4 g (6%)
Saturated Fat 1 g (5%)
Trans Fat 0 g
Monounsaturated Fat 1 g
Cholesterol 119 mg (40%)
Sodium 588 mg (25%)
Total Carbohydrates 28 g (9%)
Dietary Fiber 3 g (11%)
Sugars 1 g
Protein 33 g
Vitamin A (3%)
Vitamin C (3%)
Calcium (7%)
Iron (16%)

*Parenthetical percentages refer to % Daily Value.

Fried chicken or fish doesn't have to be deep-fat-fried to have all the flavor. This recipe works well with any piece of chicken (with or without the bone). Use skinless legs, thighs, or breasts.

1. Place the egg, egg white, and mustard in a small bowl. Whisk until smooth.

2. In a food processor fitted with a steel blade, place the melba toast, thyme, rosemary, oregano, garlic powder, salt, black pepper, and cayenne. Process into small crumbs. Leave some pieces about the size of currants.

3. Preheat the oven to 400°F. Dredge a chicken breast in the egg mixture, coating thoroughly. Dredge in the bread crumbs, patting and turning frequently until well coated.

4. Place the chicken on a cookie sheet or baking rack and then place in the oven. Bake for 3 minutes and then lightly spray the top of each chicken breast with the oil. Bake for 5 minutes more and then turn. Spray lightly with the oil again and bake for about 6 more minutes.

Roasted Corn on the Cob

SERVINGS: 2 ▌ SERVING SIZE: 1 EAR CORN ▌ THIS RECIPE IS EASILY MULTIPLIED ▌
COOKING TIME: 25 MINUTES

2 ears corn
¼ teaspoon salt
⅛ teaspoon freshly ground
   black pepper
2 teaspoons unsalted butter

NUTRITION FACTS

Serving size 1 ear
Servings 2
Calories 144
Calories from Fat 44
Total Fat 5 g (8%)
Saturated Fat 3 g (13%)
Trans Fat 0 g
Monounsaturated Fat 1 g
Cholesterol 10 mg (3%)
Sodium 320 mg (13%)
Total Carbohydrates 26 g (9%)
Dietary Fiber 3 g (11%)
Sugars 4 g
Protein 3 g
Vitamin A (2%)
Vitamin C (11%)
Calcium (0%)
Iron (4%)

*Parenthetical percentages
refer to % Daily Value.

1. Preheat the oven to 400°F.

2. Peel the husks back from the corn, being careful not to detach the husks from the stem. Remove the silks and rinse well, wetting down the husks.

3. Sprinkle the salt and pepper over the corn.

4. Fold the husks back down against the corn and wrap the whole cobs in foil.

5. Roast in the oven for about 30 minutes. Turn them a quarter turn every 7 to 8 minutes.

6. Remove from the oven and unwrap the foil. Cut the bottom of the cob so that the husks fall away easily.

7. Serve each with a pat of butter.

These can also be roasted on top of the grill. The heat should be medium to medium-high and you must turn them frequently, as noted above.

Dr. Tim Says . . . Corn Is a Whole Grain

I think that people often forget about corn. While it is a carbohydrate, it is also a whole grain. Those lovely kernels have everything you need—good-quality starches, vitamins, and fiber. As a starch on your dinner plate, corn is a great choice, because a medium ear contains only about 75 calories.

Pan-Grilled Broccoli

SERVINGS: 2 ▌ **SERVING SIZE:** 4 OUNCES BROCCOLI ▌ THIS RECIPE CAN BE MULTIPLIED.
THIS WILL KEEP FAIRLY WELL IF CHILLED IMMEDIATELY. ▌ **COOKING TIME:** 25 MINUTES

8 ounces broccoli spears
Spray olive oil
⅛ teaspoon salt

NUTRITION FACTS

Serving size 4 ounces broccoli
Servings 2
Calories 39
Calories from Fat 4
Total Fat <1 g (1%)
Saturated Fat 0 g (0%)
Trans Fat 0 g
Monounsaturated Fat 0 g
Cholesterol 0 mg (0%)
Sodium 44 mg (2%)
Total Carbohydrates 8 g (3%)
Dietary Fiber 3 g (12%)
Sugars 2 g
Protein 2 g
Vitamin A (14%)
Vitamin C (169%)
Calcium (5%)
Iron (5%)

*Parenthetical percentages
refer to % Daily Value.

1. Place a large ovenproof skillet or roasting pan in the oven and preheat to 400°F.

2. Trim the bottom inch of the stem from the broccoli. Using a vegetable peeler, peel the tough outer layer from the stems.

3. Heat 1 quart of water over high heat in a large saucepan or stockpot fitted with a steamer basket. When the water is boiling, place the broccoli in the steamer and cook for 12 to 15 minutes, until the spears begin to lose their firmness. Have ready a bowl filled with 2 quarts of ice water.

4. Remove the broccoli spears from the steamer and plunge into the ice water. When the spears are cooled, remove from the water and drain.

5. When the pan is hot, add the broccoli, spray lightly with olive oil, and sprinkle with the salt. Bake for about 5 minutes and turn to sear well. Make sure that all of the spears come in contact with the pan. They will take about 15 minutes total baking time and should be turned every 3 to 5 minutes.

Day 22 Alternative Dinner Choices

CONVENIENCE MEALS

Michael Angelo's Signature Line Chicken Parmesan

RESTAURANT MEALS

Applebee's Tortilla Chicken Melt

DAY 23 | THE DR. GOURMET PANTRY: MAKE A LIST OF THE VEGETABLES YOU LIKE, AND EAT THEM

Getting more veggies in your diet is one of the basics of the Mediterranean diet. The best part is that it's the one thing you can't get too much of. (It's unlikely that you'll hear your doctor say, "Hmm, my lab tests show that you've been eating too many carrots.")

Much of the research on vegetables in the diet is focused on the antioxidants abundant in everything from asparagus to zucchini. It is now clear that that you just can't get the same benefits from taking those vitamins, minerals, and antioxidants in pill form. Recent studies show no benefit from taking supplements, but getting the same vitamins from vegetables is pretty powerful[3]: each additional serving of fruit and vegetables per day reduces your risk of heart disease by 4 percent. That's huge! But it's not just about heart disease. Putting more veggies on your plate has also been shown to reduce the risk of multiple types of cancers. Plus, that research also shows a clear weight-loss benefit.

Maybe you're like my patients who say, "But I just don't like vegetables." They are quite sincere. When I ask if there are any veggies they *will* eat, I always get some sort of response. They will say, "Oh, I do like squash," or "Tomatoes and lettuce are fine." I keep asking and they keep coming up with ones that they will eat. I generally stop around seven or eight different veggies, even though they said they wouldn't eat them because they "just don't like vegetables."

This is how you should get started. Make a list. What *do* you like? After you've done that, make a list of recipes you love. For instance, my patients may say they don't like carrots, but when I ask about a particular recipe such as candied carrots, they will say, "I love those, but they're only for Thanksgiving." Of course there's no recipe that's just for a single day of the year, especially if it's veggies! Find the recipes you love, put the ingredients on your grocery list, and get what you need the next time you are at the store.

Plan on an extra helping of those veggies for dinner. Buy enough at one time to allow you to make more. It's just as easy to double the servings of green beans amandine as it is to cook a single batch. It won't add many calories and they'll fill you up. You'll be healthier and there is excellent research to show that you'll be far more satisfied.

Keep in mind that vegetables aren't just for dinner. You can pile as many veggies on your sandwich at lunch as you want: lettuce, tomatoes, cucumbers, green peppers, red peppers, onions, mushrooms, sprouts . . . The list is endless and every day your sandwich will be an adventure.

Making vegetables part of your life as snacks is another great way to eat more. There's fantastic research that shows how satisfying this can be.

Simple changes in just one of the foundation areas of a Mediterranean-style diet can have a profound impact on your weight and long-term health. Make the produce section at the grocery store your first stop.

Many of the Dr. Gourmet recipes begin with a serving or more of veggies and that's a great way for you to get more in your life. Keep onions, celery, peppers, carrots, and the like on hand so you have a great foundation for your meals.

Another good strategy is to select a new veggie each time you are in the produce section. You may have thought that you didn't like something or not know how to prepare it. Beyond the recipes in this book there are dozens at DrGourmet.com.

Eggplant Parmesan

SERVINGS: 2 ▮ **SERVING SIZE:** A LOT ▮ THIS RECIPE CAN EASILY BE MULTIPLIED ▮
COOKING TIME: 60 MINUTES ▮ THESE KEEP WELL FOR ABOUT 48 HOURS IN THE FRIDGE.
THIS IS A TIME-CONSUMING RECIPE BUT OH, SO WORTH IT!

2 (8-ounce) eggplants, cut lengthwise into ½-inch slices
2 ounces plain, no-salt-added melba toast
¼ teaspoon dried basil
¼ teaspoon dried oregano
¼ teaspoon garlic powder
⅛ teaspoon freshly ground black pepper
2 egg whites
4 ounces fresh mozzarella cheese
8 large leaves fresh basil
1 cup bottled marinara sauce (see Note on page 150)
1 ounce Parmigiano-Reggiano cheese, grated

NUTRITION FACTS

Serving size about 3 cups
Servings 2
Calories 451
Calories from Fat 155
Total Fat 18 g (27%)
Saturated Fat 10 g (49%)
Trans Fats 0 g
Monounsaturated Fat 5 g
Cholesterol 43 mg (14%)
Sodium 1,069 mg (45%)
Total Carbohydrates 45 g (15%)
Dietary Fiber 11 g (43%)
Sugars 11 g
Protein 30 g
Vitamin A (14%)
Vitamin C (24%)
Calcium (66%)
Iron (19%)

*Parenthetical percentages refer to % Daily Value.

It is something that you should probably save for a special occasion, as it will take about an hour (or a little more) to make. But it is very rewarding. Although this is a recipe that is higher in fat and sodium than many in this book, it can still be part of your diet occasionally, and it should because Eggplant Parmesan is so delicious. You can feel better because this is chock-full of great nutrients like fiber, vitamin A, iron, calcium, and vitamin C.

1. Preheat the oven to 350°F.

2. Place 1 cup of water in a large stockpot fitted with a steamer. Heat over high heat. When the water is boiling, place the eggplant slices in the steamer and steam for 10 minutes. Transfer the eggplant to a cutting board to cool.

3. While the eggplant is steaming, place the melba toast, basil, oregano, garlic powder, and pepper in a food processor or mini chopper and process until they are fine crumbs.

4. Whisk the egg whites until frothy. When the eggplant is cool, coat each slice one at a time with egg white. Let excess egg white drip off and then dredge the eggplant in the breadcrumb mixture. As each slice is coated, place on a nonstick cookie sheet.

5. Place the coated eggplant in the oven and bake for 10 minutes on each side.

[CONTINUES]

6. Remove from the oven and layer the eggplant with slices of mozzarella and fresh basil in two single-serving au gratin or similar dishes, in this order: slice of eggplant, slice of mozzarella, basil, slice of eggplant, slice of mozzarella, and so on. It's okay if the layers are on their side or not just perfect.

7. Top the eggplant layers with the marinara sauce and bake for 5 minutes. Top with the Parmigiano-Reggiano and bake for another 5 minutes. Serve.

Note: On the DrGourmet.com Web site, we review and rate bottled tomato sauces.

Day 23 Alternative Dinner Choices

CONVENIENCE MEALS

Michael Angelo's Italian Natural Cuisine Vegetable Lasagna

RESTAURANT MEALS

Souplantation/Sweet Tomatoes Joan's Broccoli Madness

DAY 24 | THE DR. GOURMET PANTRY: EAT FRUIT AND NUTS

Nuts are great for you. While they do have a lot of calories, these are the best-quality calories because they are high in monounsaturated fat. Nuts have been shown to be very satisfying and this makes them a great choice for snacking. Instead of reaching for potato chips or crackers, have nuts. There's great research that shows you won't gain weight by eating nuts, whereas eating potato chips is clearly linked with disease.[4]

Even though nuts are high in fat and calories, they are way better for you than a snack food such as Doritos. Nuts have a few more calories per ounce (170 compared to 140 for the Doritos), but about half the salt (85 mg for the nuts versus 180 mg for the Doritos). A word about sodium: You're better off eating salted nuts than junk food such as chips or crackers, but it's even better to start eating unsalted nuts rather than salted.

One important study shows that nuts added to a Mediterranean diet dramatically reduced the risk of developing metabolic syndrome (a grouping of conditions including diabetes, hypertension, and high cholesterol).[5] In another study of those already on a Mediterranean diet, adding walnuts resulted in an additional 4 percent decrease in total cholesterol. Research on almonds shows that adding 3 ounces of almonds per day to a normal diet for nine weeks resulted in as much as a 10 percent drop in cholesterol. To make it even better, nuts and seeds are chock-full of antioxidants and vitamin E, as well as magnesium, copper, plant sterols, protein, and fiber.

Even in those already eating a Mediterranean diet, increasing the amount of walnuts people ate was shown to lower total and LDL (bad) cholesterol an extra 6 percent over their already healthy diet. I love pistachios, for example, and there is a study showing the same kind of improvement in cholesterol profiles when participants ate 20 percent of their recommended calories in pistachios.[6] Studies with walnuts and almonds show similar results.

I buy nuts and seeds in bulk at a grocery store that has bulk bins, such as at Whole Foods Market, but they can also be found in a lot of health food stores. Keep your nuts sealed in zippered plastic bags or plastic containers. I always have the following on hand:

Almonds (whole, slivered, and sliced)
Peanuts (these are actually legumes, not nuts)
Pecans
Pine nuts
Pumpkin seeds (also called pepitas)
Sesame seeds (white and black)
Sunflower seeds
Walnuts

Peanut butter is a fantastic choice for lunch or snacks, and I especially love the freshly ground kind available in some stores. If you purchase peanut butter in jars, look for the ones with the fewest ingredients.

One important note for those with diverticulosis. It may be that you have been told to avoid eating nuts and seeds in the past, to prevent a flare-up of diverticulitis. Thank goodness, this has now been disproven. In fact, in a recent study, those with diverticulosis who ate more than two servings of nuts a week had about the same or slightly lower risk of flare-ups than those who ate less than one serving per month.[7] (This included popcorn, corn, and the tiny seeds from strawberries and blueberries.) So eat your nuts and seeds and enjoy them!

There is just as much proof of the benefits of eating fruit. One study[8] looked at whether an apple a day actually does keep the doctor away. Researchers in Finland were looking at the effect of diet and antioxidants on different diseases; specifically, trying to understand what types of antioxidants, such as flavonols and flavones, might offer protection against disease.

The study showed that the more apples people ate, the lower their risk of heart disease, diabetes, lung cancer, and asthma. Another group demonstrated the positive effects of apples against ongoing genetic damage. In both cases, the researchers felt that it was the high antioxidant content in apples that made the difference.

I wrote earlier about how great fiber is for you—and apples, like most fruit, have a lot of fiber (more with the peel than without). They have as much as a slice of whole wheat bread, but only about 80 calories. This makes them the perfect snack. We know that people who fall into the "sweet snacker" category are a perfect match for fruit.[9] One study showed that those folks who ate an apple were nearly as satisfied as when they ate a chocolate bar—but they felt much less guilty about eating the fruit.

Keep your fridge full of apples, grapes, oranges, pears, and other fruit so you are prepared should the urge to snack strike. Fresh fruit is a better choice than fruit juice, because eating the fruit has been shown to be much more satisfying than drinking a glass of juice. Have as much plain fruit every day as you want. As with veggies, it's hard to gain weight by eating fruit. Have fruit with meals as a dessert and for snacks when you're craving something sweet.

Eating more fruits and veggies (and less junk food) will help you be healthier. But I want you to also know about the right portion sizes. Here are some guidelines, with calorie counts. Compare these to a Hershey bar, which has 210 calories. That's the equivalent of almost three apples!

Fruit

FRUIT		
FRUIT	SERVING SIZE	CALORIES
Apple	1 (2¾-inch diameter)	77
Applesauce (sugar free)	½ cup	84
Banana	1 (6-inch long)	90
Blackberries	1 cup	62
Blueberries	1 cup	84
Cantaloupe	¼ large melon	69
Cherries	15	77
Cranberries (dried/sweetened)	¼ cup	92
Cranberries (fresh)	2 cups	94
Currants (dried)	¼ cup	102
Grapefruit	1 cup sections	74
Honeydew melon	⅙ large melon	86
Mandarin oranges	¾ cup	78
Mango	¾ cup	80
Orange	3 inch diameter	86
Papaya	1½ cups	82
Pineapple	1 cup	82
Plums	1 cup	76
Raisins	¼ cup	15
Raspberries	¾ cup	96
Strawberries	¾ cup	73
Watermelon	2 cups	92

I am not a fan of fruit juices. I think that it's fine to have juice every now and then, but keep in mind that the calories are not going to be as satisfying as the fruit itself.

JUICES		
FRUIT	SERVING SIZE	CALORIES
Apple	1 cup	112
Cranberry	1 cup	116
Grape	1 cup	128
Grapefruit	1 cup	101
Orange	1 cup	110
Prune	½ cup	91

Nuts

Research shows you won't gain weight having nuts instead of processed snack foods. That said, they contain a lot of calories and even though they are great-quality calories you want to be cautious.

NUTS AND SEEDS		
NUTS/SEEDS	SERVING SIZE	CALORIES
Almonds	¼ cup	206
Cashews	¼ cup	187
Peanuts	¼ cup	205
Pecans	¼ cup	188
Pine nuts	¼ cup	227
Pistachios	¼ cup	171
Pumpkin seeds	¼ cup	187
Sunflower seeds	¼ cup	67
Walnuts	¼ cup	191

Shrimp Fried Rice

SERVINGS: 2 ▮ SERVING SIZE: ABOUT 2½ CUPS FRIED RICE ▮ THIS RECIPE CAN EASILY BE
MULTIPLIED ▮ THIS RECIPE MAKES GREAT LEFTOVERS ▮ COOKING TIME: 30 MINUTES

½ cup uncooked brown rice
2 teaspoons sesame oil
1 medium-size white onion,
    diced
2 large carrots, peeled and
    diced
1 rib celery, diced
⅔ cup frozen peas, thawed
6 ounces shrimp, peeled,
    deveined, and sliced in
    half lengthwise
Freshly ground black
    pepper
4 teaspoons low-sodium soy
    or tamari sauce
1 large egg, beaten

NUTRITION FACTS

Serving size about 2½ cups
    fried rice
Servings 2
Calories 434
Calories from Fat 90
Total Fat 10 g (16%)
Saturated Fat 2 g (10%)
Trans Fat 0 g
Monounsaturated Fat 4 g
Cholesterol 233 mg (78%)
Sodium 577 mg (24%)
Total Carbohydrates 57 g (19%)
Dietary Fiber 7 g (28%)
Sugars 9 g
Protein 28 g
Vitamin A 21 (4%)
Vitamin C (33%)
Calcium (13%)
Iron (25%)

*Parenthetical percentages
refer to % Daily Value.

This is a perfect weeknight meal and so much better for you than getting Asian takeout. You will save up to 500 calories per serving by making this yourself.

In the time it takes to drive to the Chinese restaurant, you can make this recipe. To make it even easier, purchase precut veggies at the market and buy the shrimp already peeled and deveined. Use instant brown rice; we have tested it in the Dr. Gourmet kitchens and it works well—especially for this sort of recipe. (Instant white rice, on the other hand, is terrible.)

1. Place 2½ cups of water in a small saucepan over high heat. When the water boils, add the rice and lower the heat to a simmer.

2. Cook, partially covered, until the water cooks away. Do not stir the rice. When cooked, remove from the stove and let cool.

3. When ready to cook, place the sesame oil in a wok or large skillet over high heat. When the oil is nearly smoking, add the onion, carrots, and celery. Cook for 3 to 4 minutes, until the onion begins to soften.

4. Add the peas and shrimp. Cook until the shrimp is pink, stirring frequently. Add the pepper to taste and the soy sauce.

5. Add the cooked rice and toss until the rice, veggies, and shrimp are well blended. Let the rice rest for at least 45 seconds so that the pan reheats. Toss again.

6. Add the beaten egg and toss until the egg is cooked through. Serve.

Day 24 Alternative Dinner Choices

CONVENIENCE MEALS

Lean Cuisine Salmon with Basil

RESTAURANT MEALS

Red Lobster Garlic-Grilled Jumbo Shrimp

COMMON FISH AND SHELLFISH

FISH/SHELLFISH	MERCURY (PPM)	OMEGA-3 FATS (MGS)
Golden bass (Gulf of Mexico)	1.45	905
Shark	0.99	689
Swordfish	0.98	819
King mackerel	0.73	401
White tuna (albacore)	0.35	862
Lobster	0.31	84
Halibut	0.25	465
Snapper	0.19	321
Mahi-mahi	0.15	139
Mussels	<0.15	782
Golden bass (Atlantic)	0.14	905
Light tuna	0.12	270
Atlantic cod	0.1	158
Crab	0.09	351
Trout	0.07	935
Atlantic mackerel	0.05	1203
Farmed salmon	<0.05	2648
Anchovy	<0.05	2055
Atlantic herring	<0.05	2014
Wild salmon	<0.05	1043
Sardines	<0.05	982
Oysters	<0.05	688
Scallops	<0.05	365
Shrimp	<0.05	315
Clams	<0.05	284
Farmed catfish	<0.05	177

DAY 25 | *THE DR. GOURMET PANTRY: EAT CEREALS AND WHOLE GRAINS*

Increasing whole grains and cereals in your diet has an amazing range of benefits, likely due to an increased fiber intake. In one study,[11] men who ate more fiber had a far lower risk of weight gain over time: up to 48 percent lower for the highest intake of fiber. For women, the effect was not as dramatic, but those eating the most fiber still had a decreased risk of weight gain of 19 percent.

The benefits extend well beyond weight control, however. Eating more whole grains has been shown to lower total and LDL cholesterol, reduce blood pressure, and prevent heart disease. And it doesn't take a major change. One study showed that having only about two slices of whole-grain bread per day had a major impact. The difference in reduction in risk of heart attack was major with a 21 percent lower risk in those eating more whole grains.[12]

I think that the best advice that I can give to folks for changing their diet is to try to eat foods that have been processed as little as possible. This is most true with grains or cereals. For instance, if you are going to have cereal for breakfast, the more basic the cereal is, the better. Oatmeal is better than shredded wheat or Cheerios, which are better than corn flakes. All of these are better than sugared cereals such as Frosted Flakes or Froot Loops (but you already knew that). Use the 20/5 rule here. Look at the Nutrition Facts box and choose a cereal with higher fiber and lower sugar.

When looking at other ingredients, remember that brown is better than white.

If you are used to eating white bread, make the transition slowly. You'll find "light" whole wheat breads in the grocery that taste great. They are not as high in fiber as regular whole wheat bread, but this is a great place to start moving yourself toward whole-grain breads. Once you have made the transition, you will find a wide variety of baked goods, including whole wheat hamburger buns, whole-grain waffles, and whole wheat pizza crust.

Whole wheat pasta is another easy change to make, and you'll find that it gives a whole new flavor to your pasta dishes. What's really interesting is that whole wheat pasta is actually the more authentic product. Refining flour strips away the fiber and nutrients; "white" pasta is a relatively new creation. When all that goodness is taken away, so is most of the richness of flavor.

The same is true of brown rice. Like whole wheat pasta, this is one of the easiest changes to make to increase your fiber intake. Brown rice takes a little longer to cook and requires more water (generally about half again as much as when cooking white rice). Wild rice is another great choice, with tons of fiber, and even better, lots and lots of flavor. In almost any recipe that calls for rice you can also substitute bulgur wheat or quinoa. Both go well in soups and are wonderful for making salads.

Lastly, people don't think of corn as a whole grain, but it is, and fresh or even frozen corn is a great option. Snacking on popcorn is also a great way to increase your intake of whole grains.

Look to include as many whole grains on your shopping list as you can; they're perfect products for your cupboard or fridge.

So what are the best-quality carbs for your new pantry?

1. Whole Grain Bread. Bread is a great place to start because so many people fear it. Don't. Bread is a great part of a healthy diet. The key is to choose whole-grain breads and look for the highest fiber. A slice of white bread has little nutritive value, with sometimes less than 1 gram of fiber. Look for breads with at least 2 grams of fiber or more per slice.

2. Whole Wheat Pasta. The other carb that people love to hate is pasta. The issue is not that pasta makes people gain weight, but that too much of a good thing is just that: too much. A serving of any pasta is 2 ounces (not half the box). Choosing whole wheat pasta is a quick and easy way to get better-quality carb calories. As with bread, the difference in fiber is almost double. There are less than 2 grams of fiber in 2 ounces of regular pasta, but almost 5 grams of fiber in the same amount of whole wheat pasta.

3. Brown Rice. The same holds true for rice. I occasionally use white rice in some dishes, such as risottos, but I love brown rice. You'll find that there are a lot of varieties of brown rice in the market now. You can easily find brown long-grain and short-grain, basmati, and jasmine rice. Almost any of your recipes that call for white rice work well with brown rice; just be sure to adjust the cooking time.

4. High-Fiber, Low-Sugar Cold Cereals and Oatmeal. Choosing a breakfast cereal is a bit like choosing whom to marry: for most of us, it has to be just right. The key is to look for cereals that are higher in fiber and lower in sugar. It really is just that simple. It is easy to figure out that sugared cereals are bad for you. Your best strategy in choosing among the others will be to look carefully at the package, try different cereals and keep the best quality in your pantry.

Breakfast cereals such as oatmeal or Cheerios are low in sugar and high in fiber. If you have a sweet tooth, you're better off sprinkling a teaspoon of sugar on your cereal, because that's only 4 grams of carbs (about 16 calories). Compare that to some raisin brans that have both added sugar *and* high-fructose corn syrup, which has 19 grams of carbohydrate per serving.

Start by looking at the amount of fiber, and, as always, the higher the better. Do just the opposite with sugar: Choose the lowest. But don't stop there—look at the ingredient list. If there's sugar, high-fructose corn syrup, or honey anywhere in the ingredient list, it's best to think twice. Certainly if any sugar ingredient is listed among the first three, it's best to leave it on the shelf.

5. Potatoes and Sweet Potatoes. Another starch that folks want to avoid is potatoes. This is a real shame. Fresh potatoes are a great example of quality calories. As with pasta, the problem is not that potatoes make you gain weight or that they are bad for you, but that people just plain eat too much (and mostly in the form of greasy French fries or potato chips). A serving of potatoes is no more than about 6 ounces, but some Idaho baking potatoes can weigh almost three times as much. Another great choice is to have yams or sweet potatoes instead. They are lower in calories and have two-thirds more fiber.

As with many considerations for eating healthy, choosing the best ingredients—the best-quality calories—is the way to success. You don't have to cut out carbs altogether; just watch the portion size and select the best quality.

Here's how to make quick changes for you:

INSTEAD OF EATING . . .	TRY EATING . . .	SERVING SIZE
White bread	Whole wheat bread	1 slice
English muffin	Whole wheat English muffin or whole grain waffles	1 muffin
Regular pasta	Whole wheat pasta	2 ounces
Potatoes	Yams or sweet potatoes	4 ounces
White rice	Brown rice	¼ cup (uncooked)
White rice	Corn	1 medium-size ear ⅔ cup frozen
White rice	Quinoa	¼ cup (uncooked)
White rice	Barley	¼ cup (uncooked)
White rice	Wild rice	¼ cup (uncooked)
Grits	Oatmeal	⅓ cup (uncooked)
Sugared cereal (e.g., Froot Loops)	100% Bran Cheerios Kashi Cinnamon Harvest Kashi GoLean Kellogg's All Bran Kellogg's Special K Shredded Wheat & Bran Total Raisin Bran Total Whole Grain Grits Quinoa	1 cup
Fruit juice	Fresh fruit	

AVOID THESE	AND EMBRACE THESE
Candy bar	Fresh fruit, smoothies
Cookies	Fresh fruit
Cake	Fresh fruit
Potato chips	Popcorn
Crackers	Nuts, peanut butter
Soda	Iced tea
Soda	Coffee
Soda	Water

Spring Barley Salad

SERVINGS: 3 ▌ **SERVING SIZE:** ABOUT 2 CUPS ▌ THIS RECIPE CAN EASILY BE MULTIPLIED ▌ **COOKING TIME:** 60 MINUTES ▌ THIS RECIPE MAKES VERY GOOD LEFTOVERS

1 cup pearled barley
1 small shallot, minced
2 ribs celery, diced
2 medium-size carrots, peeled and diced
1 medium-size yellow summer squash, seeded and diced
½ medium-size green bell pepper, seeded and diced
4 radishes, sliced very thinly
2 ounces feta cheese, crumbled
2 tablespoons pine nuts
2 tablespoons capers
2 tablespoons liquid from capers
6 large leaves fresh basil, cut in chiffonade
3 tablespoons olive oil
¼ teaspoon salt
Freshly ground black pepper

NUTRITION FACTS

Serving size about 2 cups
Servings 3
Calories 454
Calories from Fat 175
Total Fat 20 g (31%)
Saturated Fat 5 g (25%)
Trans Fat 0 g
Monounsaturated Fat 11 g
Cholesterol 17 mg (6%)
Sodium 630 mg (26%)
Total Carbohydrates 61 g (20%)
Dietary Fiber 13 g (52%)
Sugars 4 g
Protein 11 g
Vitamin A (146%)
Vitamin C (38%)
Calcium (15%)
Iron (14%)

*Parenthetical percentages refer to % Daily Value.

Barley makes a great alternative to pasta or rice salads. It has a terrific, slightly chewy texture that goes well in a salad like this one. You could substitute barley for pasta or rice in your favorite salad. The rule of thumb is 1 cup of uncooked barley = 3 servings. Likewise, you're not stuck with the veggies in this salad. Like asparagus or spinach? Add that instead of the peppers and squash.

1. Place 2 quarts of water in a large stockpot over high heat. When it begins to boil, add the barley and lower the heat to medium-high, so that the barley is at a slow rolling boil. Stir occasionally.

2. While the barley is cooking, place the shallot, celery, carrots, squash, bell pepper, radishes, feta cheese, pine nuts, capers, caper liquid, and basil in a large bowl. Fold together gently.

3. Add 2 tablespoons of the olive oil to the bowl and fold together gently. Place the bowl in the refrigerator.

4. When the barley is just cooked (about 20 minutes), it will be slightly firm and chewy, but it won't have a grainy texture. Drain and place in a second bowl. Add the remaining tablespoon of olive oil and fold gently. Let the barley cool for about 10 minutes and then put it in the refrigerator to chill.

5. After about 30 minutes, fold the chilled barley into the bowl with the veggies, and add the salt and pepper to taste. Chill for another 30 minutes or so, then serve.

Dr. Tim Says . . . Eat Barley

Barley is one of the oldest cultivated cereal grains and is perfect for soups, stews, and casseroles. It has long been used in brewing beer and making whiskey, but it has also been a popular starch in many cultures. Unfortunately, it has not remained as popular as rice, pasta, or potatoes, even though it is amazingly good and healthy—in many ways better than other starches.

Barley must have its outer hull stripped away to make it edible. The form that is available in most groceries is pearled barley, which has been hulled and then processed to remove the bran. In the process it is polished, resulting in a pearly sheen.

Barley (even if pearled) has a ton of fiber. A quarter cup of cooked barley has 8 grams of fiber. There's great research that barley will lower LDL cholesterol (bad cholesterol) and stabilize blood sugars in diabetics. The beta-glucan fiber found in barley is similar to that found in oat bran, beans, and peas. As a result, the U.S. government now allows a health claim on barley that it lowers cholesterol.

Dehulled barley is also made into a variety of other products, including flour and cereals similar to oatmeal and grits. Hulled barley is more nutritious because the bran layer has not been polished off, but it can be more difficult to find. You might find it listed as barley "groats." It will take longer to cook than pearled barley, however. When raw, barley looks like a cross between orzo pasta and wheat berries. After cooking, it has a lovely, nutty flavor.

Chef Tim Says . . . How to Make a Chiffonade

In French, this means "made of rags," so slicing a food into very thin strips is known as a *chiffonade*. Lining up the leaves of spinach and slicing across, yielding long thin strips, is a chiffonade. This is also done with herbs, such as basil or mint, by stacking the leaves, rolling them up in a tube, and cutting across the roll into ribbons.

Day 25 Alternative Dinner Choices

CONVENIENCE MEALS

Healthy Choice Tomato Basil Penne

RESTAURANT MEALS

Wendy's Broccoli and Cheese Potato

The word *legume* refers not only to the species of plants, but also to any fruit that grows seeds lined up in a pod. (I find it interesting that peas and black beans are actually considered to be fruit.) Also known as pulses, legumes are categorized as beans, lentils, peas, peanuts, snap beans, and edible pods. They're full of protein and fiber, but most of their calories come from carbohydrates. Because they are starches, it's easy to make them part of your meals, replacing pasta, rice, or potatoes.

These little guys can be one of the most powerful changes you can make in your diet. One study of ten thousand men and women showed that eating just one serving of lentils or chickpeas each week reduced the risk of heart disease.[13] And the more you eat, the more you reduce your risk. Eating legumes four or more times per week reduced the risk of heart disease by 22 percent. Twenty-two percent! That's huge! And all you have to do is have a peanut butter sandwich for lunch (remember, peanuts are legumes).

We also know that soybeans and soy products reduce the risk of both heart disease and cancers. There has been controversy about whether soy might increase the risk of breast cancer in women, but recent research shows that this is not the case. It may be that more soy in the diet actually helps to prevent breast cancer. We know this is true for other cancers as well. One study showed that those who ate the most beans had 65 percent fewer colon polyps and 50 percent fewer colon cancers.[14]

This is one change that's really easy to make part of your life. Snacking on peanuts and having peanut butter sandwiches for lunch are easy ways to add more legumes to your diet. Chili in all its endless varieties and soups such as split pea, navy bean, and black bean are really easy to make. Keep frozen peas in your freezer, as well as cans of beans in the pantry, and you'll always have enough to get more than four servings per week.

Any and all of these are great choices of legumes for you to have on hand. Note that a lot of these keep well dried or canned. When choosing canned, look for the no-salt-added versions.

Peas:

Black-eyed peas

English peas

Beans:

Black beans (turtle beans, Mexican black beans, Spanish black beans)

Cranberry beans

Fava beans (broad beans, butter beans, Windsor beans, English beans)

Flageolets

Garbanzo beans (chickpeas)

Great northern beans

Lima beans

Navy beans (Yankee beans, Boston beans, Boston navy beans)

Pinto beans

Red beans

Red kidney beans (Mexican beans, red beans)

Soybeans (edamame, soya beans)

White kidney beans (cannellini beans, fazolia beans)

Snap Beans:

Chinese long beans

French green beans (haricots verts)

Green beans (string beans)

Runner beans (Italian flat beans)

Wax beans

Edible Pods:

Okra

Snow peas (Chinese peas, Chinese snow peas)

Sugar snap peas (snap peas)

Peanuts:

Raw

Dry roasted (unsalted)

Peanut butter

Lentils:

Black lentils

Brown lentils

French green lentils (Puy lentils, *lentilles du Puy*)

Pink lentils (red lentils, *masoor dal*)

Red lentils

Yellow lentils (*moong dal*)

Seared Salmon and Chickpea Salad

SERVINGS: 4 ▌ **SERVING SIZE:** ABOUT 2 CUPS ▌ THIS RECIPE CAN EASILY BE MULTIPLIED
▌ **COOKING TIME:** 45 MINUTES ▌ THIS RECIPE MAKES GREAT LEFTOVERS

Spray olive oil
16 ounces salmon fillet
2 large carrots, peeled and
diced
2 ribs celery, diced
½ large green bell pepper,
diced
2 medium-size yellow
summer squash,
seeded and diced
2 (15-ounce) cans no-salt-
added-chickpeas,
drained and rinsed
1 teaspoon paprika
1 teaspoon dried mint
1 teaspoon dried oregano
½ teaspoon salt
Freshly ground black
pepper
1 tablespoon olive oil
1 tablespoon white wine
vinegar

NUTRITION FACTS

Serving size about 2 cups
Servings 4
Calories 456
Calories from Fat 147
Total Fat 17 g (26%)
Saturated Fat 3 g (13%)
Trans Fat 0 g
Monounsaturated Fat 8 g
Cholesterol 70 mg (23%)
Sodium 395 mg (14%)
Total Carbohydrates 8 g (3%)
Dietary Fiber 12 g (49%)
Sugars 8 g
Protein 36 g
Vitamin A (135%)
Vitamin C (36%)
Calcium (11%)
Iron (27%)

*Parenthetical percentages
refer to % Daily Value.

Two of the healthiest ingredients come together in a simple, easy salad: fiber from the veggies and legumes and rich, great-quality fat from the salmon. To make this recipe even better, choose fresh herbs.

1. Place a large ovenproof skillet in the oven and preheat the oven to 425°F. When the skillet is hot, spray the pan lightly with olive oil and add the salmon, skin side down.

2. Cook for 4 to 5 minutes and then turn. Cook for another 4 to 5 minutes and remove from the oven. Transfer to a plate and let cool for about 5 minutes. Place the plate in the fridge.

3. While the salmon is cooling, mix together the carrots, celery, green pepper, squash, chickpeas, paprika, mint, oregano, salt, and pepper to taste. Place in the fridge to chill.

4. After about 15 minutes, remove the salmon from the refrigerator and peel off the skin. Cut the skin into thin strips. Add the strips to the salad and fold. Flake the salmon into medium-size pieces. Add the flaked salmon to the salad. Fold gently.

5. Add the olive oil and vinegar and fold gently. Chill.

Chef Tim Says . . . Eat Salmon

When you step up to the fish counter, the salmon you find won't necessarily be clearly labeled. You can, however, fairly easily tell a lot about it. First, salmon is divided into two broad categories—Atlantic and Pacific.

Atlantic salmon is a species unto itself (*Salmo salar*). Wild Atlantic salmon are found in the waters of the North Atlantic, along the coast of the United States to the coasts of Europe, the United Kingdom, Iceland, and Russia. They migrate to the ocean waters of Greenland and after hanging out for a year or more near Greenland, return home to the rivers of their origin. By then, they vary in size and flavor, their pink flesh coming from a diet mostly of small crustaceans.

Because many rivers in New England are now blocked to migrating salmon, wild Atlantic salmon now run only in a very few Maine rivers. Some Atlantic salmon have, as a result, become landlocked and make their migration from deep cold water lakes into warmer tributary streams.

Atlantic salmon will generally be lighter pink in color than most Pacific varieties. It is less common to find wild Atlantic fish in markets, as most of the species is now being farmed. The majority of Atlantic salmon sold today is farm raised in Maine, Canada, and Washington state. Scotland, Norway, and Chile are also major producers. Farm-raised salmon is higher in omega-3 fats, with a 4-ounce serving having about 3,000 milligrams (mg). Wild salmon will vary but has generally less than half the amount (about 1,200 mg in 4 ounces). There is some controversy because farmed salmon has been shown to contain more pollutants. But although mercury is a concern in many fish, this is not as much of an issue with salmon.

Pacific salmon is a wholly different species and there are five types: Chinook, coho, sockeye, chum, and pink. Pacific salmon is not farmed to the extent that Atlantic salmon is.

Chinook is also known as king salmon and is a large fish with dark red flesh. Many people feel that this is the best quality of the wild salmons, with its high fat content and rich, wild flavor. I particularly like coho salmon (also called silver salmon). The flesh is not as dark as king salmon and the flavor is softer, but it still has a wonderful wild salmon taste. Small, pan-size cohos are a lighter pink and their flavor is even more subtle than other salmon varieties.

Much of the wild salmon available is sockeye. It is usually a dark pink color and early in the season is the best time to buy it. Both chum and pink salmon are widely available and these are commonly canned. They are much leaner and don't have as much flavor, but the wild fish caught early in the season, which begins in June, can be quite good.

Wild salmon contains the industrial pollutant PCBs in amounts under 5 ng/g. While this is far less than farmed fish, the amount of dioxins are similar between wild and farmed fish.

The best way to begin enjoying salmon is to start with Atlantic salmon. With its milder flavor, this fish appeals to more people than its wild Pacific cousins. After a while, begin using wild salmon in your recipes. You'll be happy with the results.

CONVENIENCE MEALS

Lean Cuisine Lemon Pepper Fish

RESTAURANT MEALS

Souplantation/Sweet Tomatoes Tuna Tarragon

DAY 27 | THE DR. GOURMET PANTRY: EAT FISH

Eat more fish and less meat. It's that simple.

Much of the research on the benefits of fish stem from research on Inuit natives and their high consumption of salmon with a correspondingly low rate of heart disease. Over time we've come to understand that this is because they are eating fish that are high in monounsaturated fats, especially omega-3 fats.

There's lots of research on the power of fish to prevent heart disease. This means fatty fish or "dark fish" such as tuna, salmon, sardines, swordfish, mackerel, or bluefish, which are all high in omega-3 fatty acids. There is even evidence that the salmon you'll have for dinner tonight can treat heart disease! A study compared 229 women who had already been diagnosed with heart disease. Researchers tracked whether the participants ate two or more servings of any kind of fish each week (or one or more serving of dark fish). After three years, the results showed that for those who ate more fish, their heart disease progressed less than those who ate less fish.[15]

We also have evidence that eating fish is good for many health problems, such as osteoporosis and infections. Fish even has a major role in the prevention of cancers, including kidney, skin, and colon cancers.[16]

The old adage that "fish is brain food" is also true. One study, for example, reported that a single meal of fish per week reduced the normal age-related decline in intelligence by 10 to 13 percent. This is the equivalent of being three or four years younger mentally. In another study, scientists looked at fish consumption as it relates to loss of memory. Those who did not eat fish had a decline four times the rate of those eating fish twice a week or more.[17]

Just as with vegetables, I have lots of patients who say that they just don't like fish. As with vegetables, make a list of those fish (or shellfish) that you do like (chances are it will be longer than you might think), and then look for healthy recipes. Even if you don't like stronger-tasting fish (e.g., tuna and salmon), freshwater fish, which are lighter tasting, may appeal to you. While leaner freshwater fish such as trout, bass, and whitefish, and shellfish such as crab, shrimp, and scallops may not be the best source of omega-3 and omega-6 fatty acids, they do contain those good fats. They're also delicious and low in calories and saturated fat.

As noted earlier, make eating fish part of your meal plans at least twice a week.

I purchase fresh seafood whenever possible. It's much easier than it used to be, given how fast ingredients can be transported, but there are a lot of good choices in the freezer case. Don't hesitate to purchase frozen fish if that's all there is available. Much of it is frozen very quickly after being caught and is "fresher" sometimes than what you might get at the fish counter.

So what should you buy? The best strategy is to go to your market, select the best fish available, and then go home to find a recipe that works, rather than choosing poor-quality fish. (This is a good reason for building the right pantry—always having the other ingredients to build your recipe.)

Let's take a look at fish that are generally easy to find and are really versatile.

Fish

If you are not used to eating fish, here's a list to get started with:

Fish especially high in monounsaturated fats:

Bluefish	Grouper	Halibut	Mackerel
Salmon	Shark	Swordfish	Tuna
Yellowtail			

You can use the following somewhat interchangeably, but some have a higher fat content and will cook somewhat differently than those listed previously.

Cod	Drum	Flounder	Mahi-mahi
Perch	Rockfish	Sea bass	Sole

Freshwater fish are good choices but don't have the same high levels of monounsaturated fats.

Catfish	Tilapia	Trout

Preparing fish can be so quick and so simple. When you're tired and you don't have time, fish for dinner is a great choice. I don't even have to write you a recipe, just some guidelines:

Preheat the oven to 375°F and place a large ovenproof skillet on the middle rack.

Sprinkle each 4-ounce fillet with about ⅛ teaspoon of salt and then some ground pepper if you like.

When the oven is hot, spray the skillet with oil and then place the fish in the pan. Lower the heat to 325°F.

After it has cooked for about 4 minutes on one side, turn the fish and drizzle about a teaspoon of olive oil over the top. Sprinkle ¼ to ½ teaspoon of your favorite herb over the top.

In another 4 minutes or so, dinner is done. Squeeze a little lemon or a splash of vinegar over the top and you are ready to eat! You can't order from Domino's in that time.

Shellfish

Sea Scallops: Sea scallops are succulent, meaty, and very satisfying. They are low in calories, with a 4-ounce serving of scallops having only 100 calories and essentially no fat.

Select large, round scallops with a translucent creamy or even pinkish color. It's best to look for "chemical free" or "day boat scallops," because treated scallops have a bitter flavor.

Bay Scallops: Bay scallops are smaller cousins to sea scallops, but there's a big difference in their flavor. Bay scallops are sweeter tasting.

The bay scallops you'll find at the fish counter are actually calico scallops. Most of the true bay scallops were killed off by a toxic alga in the 1980s, making bay scallops from Nantucket quite expensive. What you will find now are mostly from the coast of Florida and the Gulf of Mexico, and it's likely that those bay scallops have been frozen. Ask at what point they were frozen—the best ones will have been frozen on the boat, if they have been frozen at all. Choose them in the same way as you would sea scallops, looking for the same color and texture.

Mussels: Virtually all of the mussels in stores today are farmed. These are inexpensive and are very quick and easy to make.

Mussels, like clams, need to be kept ice cold and are often mishandled by markets. If the other fish at the counter don't look fresh, don't buy the mussels, either. Tightly closed shells mean the mussels are likely fresher, whereas an open shell indicates that the mussel might be dead. Don't purchase mussels with chipped or broken shells.

You can use mussels in almost any dish where you might use clams or oysters.

Clams are also low in calories and fat. I love steamed clams, but they're also great in soups, chowders, and stews.

Clams are of two varieties: Hard-shell clams and soft-shell. There are several subvarieties, which are determined primarily by where they grow as well as on the size of the clams (measured as the diameter of the shell). East Coast hard-shell clams include (smallest to largest) littleneck (<2 inches), cherrystone (a little larger, at about 2½ inches), and the quahog, a.k.a. large or chowder clam (3 inches).

The most notable West Coast hard-shell clam is the pismo (found on Pismo Beach). The small butter clam found farther north in Puget Sound is small and very tender. Soft-shells found on the West Coast include the razor clam (there is an East Coast clam called razor, but this is not a true razor clam) and the geoduck clam (pronounced *gooeyduck*). The latter is a large six-inch clam that can have a neck as long as two feet.

When buying hard-shell clams, tap each shell and the clam should close. If it doesn't, consider it dead. Soft-shell clams should retract and move a bit when the protruding neck is touched.

Shrimp: Since I now live near the Gulf, I make shrimp at least a couple of times each month. I get questions through the Web site about shrimp and cholesterol all the time. Yes, they do contain a lot of cholesterol, but as I have said before, cholesterol is not the problem, saturated fat is. Shrimp are very low in fat.

Depending on where you live, most of the shrimp that you'll buy at the fish counter have been frozen and thawed. As with the bay scallops, ask when. You can keep shrimp in your freezer for a quick meal and it'll be as good as most of the shrimp you could buy fresh at the market. Put the frozen shrimp in the refrigerator the morning you plan to make it for dinner and it'll be ready to cook when you get home.

Crab: People love eating fresh crabs, but I am not really one of them because I don't really like fighting with my food. I prefer to buy crabmeat and let someone else do the work. You'll find it sold in a variety of forms, but crabmeat will keep for only a few days in your refrigerator. Flaked crab is less expensive and comes from smaller bits of both dark and light meat from the claws and body. Lump crab is whole pieces of crab claws and the white body meat, and makes great crab cakes.

Much of what you will find on your supermarket's shelves has been pasteurized and packed in cans. This will keep about twelve to eighteen months, but the flavor is not often fresh tasting at all, so it's best to look for fresh.

Crustaceans such as crabs, crawfish, and lobster have cholesterol, just like shrimp, but also like shrimp they are very low in calories and saturated fat.

DAY 27 | DINNER

OVEN-FRIED FISH WITH YAM HOME FRIES AND PAN-GRILLED ASPARAGUS

Oven-Fried Fish

SERVINGS: 4 | **SERVING SIZE:** 1 (4-OUNCE) PIECE OF FISH | THIS RECIPE CAN EASILY BE MULTIPLIED BY 2, 3, OR 4 | THIS RECIPE CAN EASILY BE HALVED BY USING ¼ CUP OF EGG SUBSTITUTE IN PLACE OF THE EGG AND EGG WHITE | **COOKING TIME:** 60 MINUTES | LEFTOVERS KEEP WELL FOR 2 DAYS. ALLOW TO COOL BEFORE REFRIGERATING.

4 (4-ounce) fish fillets (e.g., tilapia, cod, whiting)
1 large egg
1 large egg white
1 tablespoon Dijon mustard
1 (5-ounce) box plain melba toast
¼ teaspoon salt
½ teaspoon freshly ground black pepper
Spray oil

NUTRITION FACTS

Serving size 1 fish fillet
Servings 4
Calories 258
Calories from Fat 29
Total Fat 3 g (5%)
Saturated Fat 1 g (4%)
Trans Fat 0 g
Monounsaturated Fat 1 g
Cholesterol 102 mg (34%)
Sodium 575 mg (24%)
Total Carbohydrates 28 g (9%)
Dietary Fiber 2 g (10%)
Sugars 1 g
Protein 26 g
Vitamin A (2%)
Vitamin C (2%)
Calcium (6%)
Iron (12%)

*Parenthetical percentages refer to % Daily Value.

As in the Oven-Fried Chicken recipe, the melba toast makes the coating crispy. You'll save a ton of calories over fried fish or even the frozen versions of fried fish. This recipe makes great fish sticks, too. Substitute mayonnaise for the mustard and slice the fish into strips to make this kid friendly.

1. Preheat the oven to 375°F. Place a large nonstick cookie sheet or ovenproof skillet in the oven.

2. Place the fish fillets on a stack of three paper towels so that they are not touching one another. Cover with three more paper towels and press down slightly so that as much of the fish as possible is in contact with the towels.

3. Place the egg, egg white, and mustard in a small bowl. Whisk until smooth.

4. In a food processor fitted with a steel blade, process the melba toast, salt, and black pepper until they are small crumbs. Leave some pieces about the size of currants.

5. Dredge a fish fillet in the egg mixture, coating thoroughly. Dredge in the bread crumbs, patting and turning frequently until well coated.

6. Dredge the coated fish in the egg wash a second time and then coat again with bread crumbs.

[CONTINUES]

7. Remove the pan from the oven and spray lightly with oil. Place the fish in the pan so that the fillets don't touch one another. Spray the top of the fish lightly with oil and then place in the oven. Bake for 3 minutes and then turn. Spray the top of each fillet lightly with the oil. Bake for 5 minutes more and then turn again. Spray lightly with the oil again and bake for about 6 more minutes.

8. Remove from the oven and serve immediately with tartar sauce.

Yam Home Fries

SERVINGS: 4 ▌ SERVING SIZE: ABOUT 1 CUP ▌ THIS RECIPE CAN EASILY BE DOUBLED ▌
THIS RECIPE DOES NOT MAKE VERY GOOD LEFTOVERS ▌ COOKING TIME: 30 MINUTES

1 tablespoon olive oil
1 small onion, minced
1 pound yams, peeled and
    cut into ¼- to ½-inch
    cubes
¼ teaspoon salt
Freshly ground black
    pepper
¼ teaspoon dried thyme
¼ teaspoon dried oregano

NUTRITION FACTS

Serving size 1 cup
Servings 4
Calories 169
Calories from Fat 32
Total Fat 4 g (6%)
Saturated Fat 1 g (3%)
Trans Fat 0 g
Monounsaturated Fat 3 g
Cholesterol 0 mg (0%)
Sodium 156 mg (7%)
Total Carbohydrates 33 g (11%)
Dietary Fiber 5 g (20%)
Sugars 1 g
Protein 2 g
Vitamin A (3%)
Vitamin C (34%)
Calcium (3%)
Iron (4%)

*Parenthetical percentages
refer to % Daily Value.

These Yam Home Fries are a great example of where you can use yams or sweet potatoes in place of potatoes for a great dish that's great for you.

1. Place a large ovenproof skillet in the oven and preheat the oven to 325°F.

2. When the pan is hot, place the oil, onion, and yams in the pan. Return the pan to the oven and cook for about 10 minutes. Stir the yams and continue to roast, stirring every 8 to 10 minutes. It will take about 30 minutes until the yams begin to soften.

3. Add the salt, pepper to taste, thyme, and oregano and stir. Roast for another 5 to 8 minutes, until the yams are slightly crispy on the outside and soft on the inside.

Pan-Grilled Asparagus

SERVINGS: 2 ▮ **SERVING SIZE:** 4 OUNCES ASPARAGUS ▮ THIS RECIPE CAN BE MULTIPLIED BY 4 ▮ THIS WILL KEEP FAIRLY WELL IF CHILLED IMMEDIATELY ▮ **COOKING TIME:** 15 MINUTES

8 ounces asparagus spears, woody ends removed and discarded
Spray olive oil
⅛ teaspoon salt

NUTRITION FACTS

Serving size 4 ounces asparagus
Servings 2
Calories 23
Calories from Fat 0
Total Fat 0 g (0%)
Saturated Fat 0 g (0%)
Trans Fat 0 g
Monounsaturated Fat 0 g
Cholesterol 0 mg (0%)
Sodium 153 mg (6%)
Total Carbohydrates 4 g (1%)
Dietary Fiber 2 g (10%)
Sugars 2 g
Protein 3 g
Vitamin A (17%)
Vitamin C (11%)
Calcium (3%)
Iron (14%)

*Parenthetical percentages refer to % Daily Value.

Pan-grilling asparagus brings out their natural sweetness and is so simple and easy. You can blanch the asparagus in advance (and to keep some on hand for snacking).

1. Place a large nonstick skillet or roasting pan in the oven and preheat to 400°F.

2. Heat 1 quart of water in a shallow pan over medium-high heat. The water should never come to a full boil.

3. Place the asparagus in the water and cook for 5 to 7 minutes, until the spears begin to lose their firmness. Have ready a bowl filled with 2 quarts of ice water.

4. Remove the spears from the pan and place in the ice water. When the asparagus is cooled, remove it from the water and drain.

5. When the oven skillet is hot, place the asparagus in the pan, spray lightly with olive oil, and sprinkle the salt over the top. Cook for about 5 minutes and toss the asparagus to coat well. Make sure that all sides come in contact with the pan. They will take 10 minutes total cooking time and should be tossed every 3 to 5 minutes.

CONVENIENCE MEALS

Lean Cuisine Salmon with Basil

RESTAURANT MEALS

Ruby Tuesday Asian Glazed Salmon

DAY 28 | THE DR. GOURMET PANTRY: REDUCED-FAT DAIRY

Dairy products are one of the nine elements of the traditional Mediterranean diet, but they are usually consumed in the form of processed products, such as yogurt or cheeses. Milk is not often drunk as a beverage.

Specific research on dairy is more conflicting, and much of it is funded by the National Dairy Council. The studies are often very small and in many cases appear to be biased. For instance, the Dairy Council has run an advertising campaign claiming that consuming dairy three times a day can help you lose weight. The fact is, those who increased the amount of dairy products they ate over the course of a twelve-year study[18] actually gained more weight than did those who decreased their dairy intake the most during the same period. This may be because those who ate more dairy tended to choose higher-fat dairy products, because researchers found those who ate the same amount of low-fat dairy products were much less likely to gain weight.

There have also been claims that higher calcium intake might help with weight control, but unfortunately we have proof that isn't the case, either. Even studies investigating such things as colon cancer and fat absorption in those who ate dairy products have been inconclusive. We do know that higher calcium and vitamin D consumption is important, especially for bone health, but there are many other food choices that are high in calcium.

Here are some examples of foods high in calcium:

Rice	Chickpeas	Collard greens
Crab	Halibut	Kale
Many fortified cereals	Oranges	Papayas
Peas	Raisins	Shrimp
Soybeans	Spinach	White beans

Because there's a lot of saturated fat in many dairy products, choose lower-fat milk, cheeses, and yogurts. You will find higher-fat cheeses used for recipes in this book, and you should be sure to select the best-quality cheese you can for your recipes. Parmigiano-Reggiano cheese is a more expensive ingredient than the domestic Parmesan or the stuff in the green box, but it has so much more flavor that you'll need to use much less.

Having a glass of lower-fat milk every now and then is fine, and most folks have milk on their cereal or in their coffee. You do not, however, need to eat dairy products to be healthy or for weight loss. Dairy products can be part of your life, but aim for it to be a smaller part.

If most of the dairy in the Mediterranean diet is in the form of processed products such as cheese and yogurt, what are the best choices for your fridge?

Yogurt

Much of the yogurt sold in European countries is made with lower fat and not whole milk. The same now holds true here in America, but you need will to check the package carefully. Like most dairy products, you will find whole milk yogurt at about 4 percent fat, reduced-fat at 2 percent, and nonfat yogurt.

Try to avoid yogurts that have fruit in them or are "custard style." These contain a lot of added calories because of the added sugars, often in the form of high-fructose corn syrup.

I love Greek-style yogurts. They are rich and creamy even when fat free. There are a lot of brands on the market today, so you shouldn't have trouble finding this kind.

Cheese

As with yogurt, many European cheeses are made using lower-fat milk. Such cheeses as mozzarella use skim milk, and those from goat's or sheep's milk are naturally lower in fat than those made from cow's milk.

Full-fat cheeses, however, start at around 9 grams of fat per ounce and move up from there, mostly based on how long the cheese has been aged. Cheddar is at the lower end of the fat scale, whereas an aged Parmigiano-Reggiano can be in the neighborhood of 14 grams per ounce. There are some intensely flavored cheeses with as many as 18 grams per ounce.

Even so, there are great lower-fat cheeses at the grocery. In the range of 4 to 6 grams per ounce, these include Cheddar, Swiss, and Monterey Jack. Mozzarella is a great-tasting cheese, whether it's fresh or low-moisture (like the kind you put on your pizza). The latter keeps better, and having some on hand means you're always ready to make pizza.

The nonfat cheeses you'll find on the market are terrible. They taste bad, the texture is awful, and they don't melt well. Don't bother. I use lower-fat cheeses in a lot of recipes because I find that they melt much better than their fuller-fat cousins. A regular-fat Cheddar will often separate and become oily, whereas a 6-grams-per-ounce cheese melts just right. This is not to say that you shouldn't use high-fat cheeses. Good-quality aged cheeses, such as Parmigiano-Reggiano or Romano, which are in the range of 14 grams of fat per ounce, are higher in fat but so full of flavor you can use much less.

I purchase a small amount of good-quality blue cheese and feta cheese to keep in the fridge. Blue cheese is higher in fat, but like Parmigiano-Reggiano, there's so much flavor that you only need a little. Feta cheese, like mozzarella, is naturally low in fat, but both are full of flavor.

Sour Cream

There are three types of sour cream on the market now. The regular version has 5 grams of fat per 2 tablespoons. Of this, 3.5 grams are saturated fat. There are 60 total calories, 50 of them coming from fat. I seldom use full-fat sour cream.

Reduced- or lower-fat sour cream has only 3.5 grams of fat per 2 tablespoons (2.5 of them saturated). Each serving is 45 calories. Fat-free or nonfat sour cream is just that; most of the calories are from carbohydrates.

Regular and reduced-fat sour creams can be used in cooking, but even at moderate temperatures, fat-free sour cream separates easily. I generally use the fat-free kind only for cold items, such as salad dressings.

Milk

If you are going to drink milk or use it on your cereal, use skim milk or 1%. I use 2% milk for recipes because skim or 1% milk can't offer the same creamy texture.

Buttermilk

Having buttermilk on hand is a good idea if you are going to be baking. This is no longer made fresh but is cultured and almost always uses skim milk. You can make buttermilk in a pinch by adding 1¾ tablespoons of cream of tartar or 1 tablespoon of lemon juice or white vinegar, to a cup of milk and letting it stand for 5 to 10 minutes.

Whipping Cream

I rarely use heavy cream for recipes because it's easy to get the same results using lower-fat ingredients. I like to keep canned reduced-fat whipped cream in my fridge, because I enjoy whipped cream on fresh fruit or the like, and having the can means I don't have to purchase a carton of fresh cream that will certainly go bad before I use it up.

Beef Stroganoff with Egg Noodles

SERVINGS: 6 ▌ **SERVING SIZE:** 2 CUPS ▌ THIS RECIPE CAN BE DOUBLED, BUT USE A VERY LARGE POT ▌ **COOKING TIME:** 60 MINUTES ▌ LEFTOVERS ARE GREAT. REHEAT GENTLY SO THAT THE SOUR CREAM DOESN'T BREAK DOWN.

3 tablespoons all-purpose flour
½ teaspoon freshly ground black pepper
1½ pounds flank steak, trimmed of all fat and cubed
2 teaspoons canola oil
2 medium-size onions, sliced thinly
Spray olive oil
1 pound white mushrooms, sliced
2 tablespoons freshly squeezed lemon juice
2 tablespoons Worcestershire sauce
¼ cup reduced-fat sour cream
¼ cup 2% milk
1½ tablespoons dried basil
½ teaspoon salt
2 cups low-sodium, nonfat beef or chicken stock
1 cup nonfat sour cream
12 ounces uncooked egg noodles (2 ounces per serving)

Heating reduced-fat ingredients such as reduced-fat sour cream and yogurt takes care, because they can break down and turn grainy. Heat this dish gently and you will end up with one that is as rich and creamy as the traditional. Use nonfat products later in the cooking process, so they are not overheated.

Regular and reduced-fat sour creams can be used in cooking, but even at moderate temperatures, fat-free sour cream separates easily. When adding it to hot sauces or soups, let cool first and then add the sour cream, reheating gently.

1. Preheat the oven to 350°F.

2. Place the flour and black pepper in a brown paper bag. Coat half the beef cubes by shaking them in the paper bag, remove them, and then shake the rest of the beef in the bag.

3. Place 1 teaspoon of the canola oil in a skillet and heat over medium heat. Add half of the floured beef and brown on all sides. Be careful not to let the meat touch or it will steam. As the cubes become browned on all sides, transfer to a stockpot. Repeat for the second batch of beef.

4. Brown the onion in the skillet and transfer to the stockpot. Spray the pan with oil and add the mushrooms. Cook the mushrooms until well browned, and then add them to the pot with the meat and onions.

NUTRITION FACTS

Serving size 2 cups
Servings 6
Calories 515
Calories from Fat 110
Total Fat 12 g (19%)
Saturated Fat 5 g (23%)
Trans Fats 0 g
Monounsaturated Fat 4 g
Cholesterol 57 mg (19%)
Sodium 390 mg (16%)
Total Carbohydrates 61 g (20%)
Dietary Fiber 3 g (14%)
Sugars 10 g
Protein 40 g
Vitamin A (8%)
Vitamin C (14%)
Calcium (16%)
Iron (27%)

*Parenthetical percentages refer to % Daily Value.

5. Deglaze the skillet with the lemon juice and Worcestershire. Add the deglazing liquid to the stew pot. Stir in the reduced-fat sour cream, milk, basil, salt, and beef stock until well blended. Cover the pot and place in the preheated oven. Cook for 1 hour, until the meat is tender.

6. Place 4 quarts of water in a large pot and bring to a boil. (Note: If you are going to make the full six servings [12 ounces] of beef Stroganoff, use 6 quarts of water or more in a large stockpot.) Add the appropriate amount of egg noodles (2 ounces per serving) and stir occasionally. When the noodles are cooked, drain and serve topped with the stroganoff.

7. Carefully fold the nonfat sour cream into the sauce just before serving. Serve over the noodles.

Dr. Tim Says . . .

If the label says . . .

No or Free: *Calorie-free* or *no calorie*, the product has to have less than 5 calories per serving.

No cholesterol or *cholesterol-free*, there has to be less than 2 milligrams of cholesterol in the food. Anything labeled *cholesterol-free* must also have less than 2 grams of saturated fat per serving.

When the package says *no cholesterol*, it must also tell you if it is like other foods of its type. For example, if the label says, "Corn oil margarine, a no-cholesterol food," it means that package of margarine has no cholesterol, but this is because all corn oil margarines don't have cholesterol in them.

Nonfat or Fat-free: *Nonfat* or *fat-free* foods can have no more than 0.5 gram of fat per serving. *No-fat, no added fat*, and *zero fat* mean exactly the same thing as *fat-free*.

Day 28 Alternative Dinner Choices

CONVENIENCE MEALS

Michael Angelo's Italian Natural Cuisine Lasagna with Meat Sauce

RESTAURANT MEALS

Ruby Tuesday Petite Sirloin

CHAPTER 5 | **WEEK 5 GOALS**

By now, you should have made the change to a fresher pantry and better-quality meals. You've seen that there's great research proving how much healthier you can be by making simple changes, including planning and cooking your own food. Moving forward into Week 5, you'll finish stocking your pantry as well as learn how to use it in a pinch if you get caught without something for dinner.

I have spent a lot of time talking about what you can eat. During the second half of this week we'll continue that, covering alcohol, desserts, and snacking. We'll learn about how your taste buds work and the way that you can use that knowledge to your advantage in choosing great recipes.

This week, you'll:

- Finish building your pantry with oils and learn about meats
- Learn about Dr. Gourmet pantry meals to use in a pinch
- Understand the place in your diet of alcohol, desserts, and snacks
- Learn more about the terminology used on labels
- Read about the importance of taste

A personalized shopping list for Week 5 can be found at DrGourmet.com/shoppinglist.

WEEK 5 MENU		
RECIPE	CONVENIENCE FOOD ALTERNATIVE	RESTAURANT MEAL ALTERNATIVE
DAY 29		
Seared Halibut with Basil Oil, Savory Lemon Rice, and Side Salad with Honey Mustard Dressing	Lean Cuisine Salmon with Basil	Red Lobster Garlic-Grilled Jumbo Shrimp
DAY 30		
Leftover Beef Stroganoff with Egg Noodles	Michael Angelo's Italian Natural Cuisine Lasagna with Meat Sauce	Ruby Tuesday Petite Sirloin
DAY 31		
Shrimp Enchiladas	Lean Cuisine Szechuan Style Stir Fry with Shrimp	Baja Fresh Shrimp Ensalada
DAY 32		
Portobello Burger and Spiced Snap Peas	Michael Angelo's Italian Natural Cuisine Four Cheese Lasagna	P. F. Chang's Steamed Vegetable Dumplings
DAY 33		
Paella and Crème Brûlée	Kashi Southwest Style Chicken	Baja Fresh "Baja-Style" Tacos with Chicken
DAY 34		
Baked Ziti	Healthy Choice Naturals Pumpkin Squash Ravioli	Panera Half-Serving Mediterranean Veggie Sandwich with a Fruit Cup
DAY 35		
Leftover Paella	Kashi Southwest Style Chicken	Baja Fresh Shrimp Ensalada

DAY 29 | *THE DR. GOURMET PANTRY: EAT OLIVE OIL (AND OTHER HEALTHY FATS)*

Choosing the best-quality oils and fats, and using them carefully, can have a major impact on both your health and your taste buds. Unlike in our Western diet, the primary source of fats in the Mediterranean diet is olive oil. Consequently, much of the research done on the Mediterranean diet has focused on the effects of olive oil on a person's health. That research has yielded a ton of information not just about the benefits of olive oil, but also the antioxidants and monounsaturated fats it and other vegetable oils contain.

There's a clear link between the anti-inflammatory properties of olive oil and the prevention and reversal of many diseases. Because heart disease begins with inflammatory responses in the body, adding olive oil to your diet can have a significant positive effect on heart disease, cholesterol levels, and blood pressure.[1] In fact, people who see the biggest effects are those who don't already follow a Mediterranean diet. Adding just a tablespoon a day of extra-virgin olive oil to your diet can yield an impressive reduction in blood pressure. Those who reduce the amounts of other fats they eat, to adjust for the additional fats in the olive oil, also see their cholesterol levels fall.

Less research has been done on other oils, but these positive results seem to be an effect of many seed oils—not just olive oil. One study actually showed even more improvement in cholesterol profiles when they compared grapeseed oil to olive oil.[2] There's good evidence for canola oil, as well. That said, given the overwhelming amount of research on polyphenols, flavonoids, and other antioxidants, olive oil is still probably the best bet for your diet. These sorts of antioxidant compounds have been shown to help prevent disease, including slowing the progression of heart disease, stroke, osteoporosis, cancers, and Alzheimer's disease. Avoid the more refined olive oils, as refining appears to remove some of these antioxidants and reduce the oil's positive effects.

The Mediterranean cultures do use other vegetable oils, and most cultures use some butter, but the latter is generally used sparingly. Here's a guide to choosing better oils or fats:

CHOICES FOR OILS AND FATS

GREAT CHOICES	USE WITH CARE	AVOID
Extra-virgin olive oil	Butter	Lard
Canola oil	Coconut milk	Stick margarine
Grapeseed oil	Coconut oil	Vegetable shortening (e.g., Crisco)
Safflower oil	Mayonnaise	Foods containing hydrogenated oils
Sesame oil	Spreads (e.g., Smart Balance Light and Promise Light)	Foods containing palm kernel oil
Tahini (sesame seed butter)		
Peanut butter		
Avocados		

Choosing the right oil or fat also depends on the recipe you will use it in. Olive and grapeseed oils have a fruitier flavor and are perfect for recipes where you want those tastes to come through, such as salad dressings. Use less-expensive olive oils for cooking applications, such as sautéing, and save your best-quality extra-virgin olive oil for dressings and sauces.

When you want to add less flavor, cooking with canola oil is a good choice. Sesame oil is perfect for Asian recipes; use regular for a mild taste or the dark toasted oil for a richer flavor.

As with all ingredients, be careful about measuring fats: As a rule of thumb, each teaspoon of oil, regardless of type, has about 45 calories and 5 grams of fat. This includes vegetable oils as well as butter. Low–trans fat spreads such as Smart Balance or Promise will have far fewer calories. For instance, there are only 45 calories in a tablespoon of Smart Balance, compared with the same number of calories in a teaspoon of butter.

For a lot of people, keeping a pantry full of different oils just isn't practical. Oils have a fairly short shelf life before they begin picking up odd flavors or even turning rancid. Keep just a few on hand that are versatile and healthier. Here's a guide to what to stock your new kitchen with:

Butter

Almost any unsalted butter will do. Because you won't use a lot, it's a good idea to keep it sealed in a lidded plastic container. If I buy more than a stick of butter, I freeze what I don't need right away. I do like using the higher-butterfat European-style butters because they offer a little more richness, and because I am not using all that much, it doesn't really end up costing much more in terms of price and calories.

Olive Oil

The term *cold pressed* means that the oil-refining process uses only pressure to extract the oil from the olives. After pressing, olive oils are graded based on the acidity of the oil. *Extra-virgin olive oil* is cold pressed and has 1 percent acid. Because it comes from the first pressing of the olives, it is considered the finest, having the freshest, fruitiest flavor. *Virgin olive oil* also comes from the first pressing and has about 3 percent acid.

There are other designations on olive oil labels. *Fino* is a blend of extra-virgin and virgin oil, whereas *light* means an oil that has passed through a fine filter to remove much of the sediment. Oils simply labeled *olive oil* or *pure* are a combination of refined virgin and extra-virgin oils.

I always keep extra-virgin olive oil on hand and spend a little more for the best quality, but I only use it for recipes where I want to add bright, fruity tastes, such as salad dressings. The fresh flavor and aroma of a great-quality (and usually higher-priced) oil is worth the extra money. I have less-expensive, refined virgin olive oil in the house for dishes that will lose the flavor of the oil when cooked.

Vegetable Oils

Canola oil is pressed from the rapeseed, and like olive oil, is also high in monounsaturated fat. Canola oil is pretty much flavorless and I keep it in the pantry for those recipes where I don't want to add the fruitiness of olive or grapeseed oil. It's a great choice for baking in combination with an egg yolk and/or butter.

Safflower oil is also very high in monounsaturated fat, but it's less widely available.

Grapeseed Oil

I like grapeseed oil as a middle ground between olive and canola oil. It is very high in polyunsaturated fat and studies have shown that it may be even better for you than olive oil. One study showed almost a 14 percent increase in HDL cholesterol when participants added as little as 2 tablespoons per day to their diet. In another study, 3 tablespoons of grapeseed oil, substituted for other fats in the diet, resulted in a 7 percent reduction in LDL cholesterol and a 13 percent increase in HDL levels.[3]

Here's a table to show you the comparison of the common oils on the market and the amounts of various fats they contain:

FATS			
FAT (1 TABLESPOON)	MONOUNSATURATED (G)	SATURATED (G)	POLYUNSATURATED (G)
Safflower oil	10.2	0.8	2.0
Olive oil	10.0	1.8	1.2
Canola oil	8.2	0.9	4.1
Peanut oil	6.2	2.3	4.3
Sesame oil	5.4	1.9	5.6
Corn oil	3.3	1.7	8.0
Soybean oil	3.2	2.0	7.8
Sunflower oil	2.7	1.4	8.9
Cottonseed oil	2.4	3.5	7.0
Grapeseed oil	2.2	1.3	9.5

DAY 29 | DINNER

SEARED HALIBUT WITH BASIL OIL, SAVORY LEMON RICE, AND SIDE SALAD WITH HONEY MUSTARD DRESSING

Seared Halibut with Basil Oil

SERVINGS: 2 ▓ **SERVING SIZE:** 4 OUNCES HALIBUT AND 1½ TEASPOONS BASIL OIL ▓
THIS RECIPE CAN EASILY BE MULTIPLIED ▓ **COOKING TIME:** 30 MINUTES

¼ cup extra-virgin olive oil
½ cup fresh basil leaves
2 (4-ounce) halibut fillets
¼ teaspoon salt
Freshly ground black
    pepper
Spray olive oil

NUTRITION FACTS

Serving size 4 ounces halibut
    and 1½ teaspoons basil oil
Servings 2
Calories 183
Calories from Fat 83
Total Fat 9 g (14%)
Saturated Fat 1 g (6%)
Trans Fat 0 g
Monounsaturated Fat 6 g
Cholesterol 36 mg (12%)
Sodium 351 mg (15%)
Total Carbohydrates 0 g (0%)
Dietary Fiber 0 g (0%)
Sugars 0 g
Protein 23 g
Vitamin A (5%)
Vitamin C (0%)
Calcium (6%)
Iron (6%)

*Parenthetical percentages
refer to % Daily Value.

You can use basil and herb oil as an enhancement for almost anything: salmon, cod, chicken breasts, or pork tenderloin. This is one of the quickest and easiest, yet most elegant ways to enhance your recipes because of its very simplicity.

There is no substitute for fresh basil. Dried basil has a completely different flavor and using it in recipes is something I rarely do. The fresh basil you will find in the market is most likely sweet basil. The soft green leaves bruise easily and then turn black, so fresh basil doesn't keep very well.

To keep the leaves fresh, rinse them gently and then wrap them in a damp paper towel. Place the bundle inside a plastic bag before putting them in the fridge. You can also put them stem down in a glass of water, like a bunch of flowers in a vase.

1. Place the olive oil and basil in a blender or mini chopper and process until smooth.

2. Preheat the oven to 425°F. Place a medium-size ovenproof skillet in the oven. While the oven is heating, rinse the halibut with cold water and pat dry. Place the fillets on a cutting board skin side up. Cut shallow slits in the skin about ¼ inch apart. Sprinkle the skin side of the fish with the salt and pepper.

3. When the oven is hot, spray the pan lightly with oil. Place the fish in the pan, skin side down. Return the pan to the oven and cook for 10 to 12 minutes.

4. Serve the fish skin side up, topped with 1½ teaspoons of basil oil.

Savory Lemon Rice

SERVINGS: 2 | **SERVING SIZE:** ABOUT 1 CUP | THIS RECIPE CAN EASILY BE MULTIPLIED | **COOKING TIME:** 30 MINUTES

½ cup low-sodium chicken stock
¼ teaspoon salt
1 clove garlic
½ cup uncooked brown rice
2 teaspoons lemon zest
1 tablespoon freshly squeezed lemon juice
Freshly ground black pepper

NUTRITION FACTS

Serving size 1 cup
Servings 2
Calories 185
Calories from Fat 15
Total Fat 2 g (3%)
Saturated Fat <1 g (2%)
Trans Fat 0 g
Monounsaturated Fat 1 g
Cholesterol 0 mg (0%)
Sodium 312 mg (13%)
Total Carbohydrates 38 g (13%)
Dietary Fiber 2 g (7%)
Sugars 1 g
Protein 5 g
Vitamin A (0%)
Vitamin C (12%)
Calcium (1%)
Iron (5%)

*Parenthetical percentages refer to % Daily Value.

The nutty brown rice goes well with the savory chicken stock and the zing of the lemon juice and lemon zest.

1. Place 1½ cups of water, the chicken stock and salt, and the whole clove of garlic in a medium-size saucepan over high heat.

2. When the liquid boils, stir in the brown rice, lemon zest, and lemon juice. Reduce the heat to medium-low and simmer, partially covered, for 25 to 30 minutes. Do not boil away all of the liquid and do not stir the rice.

3. When a very small amount of liquid remains, remove the pan from the burner and let it stand, covered, for about 5 minutes before serving. Remove the garlic clove and discard before serving. Add black pepper to taste.

Chef Tim Says . . . Oil Smoke Point

The temperature at which the oil will begin to smoke is called the *smoke point*. This can be important to your choice of oil because heating the oil beyond the smoke point will change its flavor (and may be less healthy). This is one of the reasons to use grapeseed oil—it has one of the higher smoke points. Here's a guide to help you:

SMOKE POINT

350°F	Butter
356°–370°F	Vegetable shortening
400°F	Canola oil
406°F	Extra-virgin olive oil
440°F	Peanut oil/Sunflower oil
450°F	Corn oil
468°F	Extra-light olive oil
485°F	Grapeseed oil

Side Salad with Honey Mustard Dressing

SERVINGS: 8 ▮ **SERVING SIZE:** 2 TABLESPOONS ▮ THIS RECIPE CAN EASILY BE MULTI-PLIED ▮ COOKING TIME: 15 MINUTES ▮ THIS RECIPE KEEPS WELL FOR ABOUT A WEEK IN THE REFRIGERATOR

1 cup fat-free sour cream
1 tablespoon coarsely
    ground mustard
2 tablespoons honey
½ teaspoon dried tarragon
2 tablespoons tarragon
    vinegar
¼ cup 2% milk
¼ teaspoon freshly ground
    black pepper

NUTRITION FACTS

Serving size 2 tablespoons
Servings 8
Calories 52
Calories from Fat 6
Total Fat 1 g (1%)
Saturated Fat 0 g (0%)
Trans Fats 0 g
Monounsaturated Fat 0 g
Cholesterol 3 mg (1%)
Sodium 49 mg (2%)
Total Carbohydrates 10 g (3%)
Dietary Fiber 0 g (0%)
Sugars 7 g
Protein 2 g
Vitamin A (4%)
Vitamin C (1%)
Calcium (6%)
Iron (1%)

*Parenthetical percentages
refer to % Daily Value.

Pair this delicious dressing with your favorite greens, but add some other veggies to it. The great thing about salad is that it's such a fantastic way to get a few extra servings of vegetables. Tear some lettuce and slice a cucumber, some celery, and green peppers. Throw on a few cherry tomatoes and you have a great side salad that's less than 125 calories with the dressing.

1. Mix all the ingredients together. If the dressing is too thick, add a small amount of milk to thin.

2. Chill for at least an hour before using.

CONVENIENCE MEALS

Lean Cuisine Salmon with Basil

RESTAURANT MEALS

Red Lobster Garlic-Grilled Jumbo Shrimp

DAY 30 | *THE DR. GOURMET PANTRY: EAT MEAT THE MEDITERRANEAN WAY*

People in Mediterranean cultures consume less meat and eat leaner meats than those in Western ones. Diet studies reveal that the former consume an average of 4 ounces or less of meat each day, so a lot of research has focused on the effect of consuming less meat.

In one study, a group who ate less lean beef or pork as part of a lower-fat diet improved their cholesterol levels in ways similar to those who ate fish or chicken instead. This appears to be because foods higher in saturated fat have a greater effect on cholesterol profiles.[4]

As with other components of the Mediterranean diet, it's not just the risk of heart disease that improves when making changes. Eating less meat and choosing meats that are lower in saturated fat are also linked to reduced cancer rates. One study showed that those who consumed high-fat and processed meats had much higher rates of colon or rectal cancer: an increase of over 40 percent.[5]

The group eating the most poultry and fish had reduced rectal cancer rates, with a decrease in risk of 19 percent, and as much as a 30 percent lower risk of other colon cancers. There have been similar results in research on meat consumption and other cancers, including breast and skin cancers. Data from the Nurses Health Study,[6] for example, showed a link between some types of breast cancers and eating more red meat. The association held true whether the measurement of red meat was in servings or by total weight consumed.

- When you are choosing meats, look for leaner cuts, as those will have less saturated fat.
- Select lean cuts of beef, such as flank steak, top round, eye of round, and London broil. Choose the leanest hamburger you can find: the lowest fat content in the grocery store. Generally this is labeled *5% fat content, 95% lean*, or *95/5*.
- Pork (also considered a red meat) can be as lean as skinless chicken. For instance, pork tenderloin or a lean pork chop has about the same calories, fat, and saturated fat as a skinless chicken breast.
- Eat red meat no more than about once a week, and poultry no more than three times over a two-week period.
- Eating skinless poultry reduces the amount of saturated fat in your meal. Cooking your chicken with the skin on, however, is just fine. Cooking the chicken without removing the skin—but then not eating the skin—doesn't add calories or saturated fat to your meal, but the chicken will be more succulent.

Bottom line? Select lean cuts of meat and enjoy them, but make them less a part of your life by eating more fish as well as more meatless meals.

Poultry

Most all of the chicken in the markets today is shipped frozen and thawed at the grocery store. Be careful of the sell-by dates on the package. There have been repeated media reports of grocery stores' repackaging and redating meats when they are close to the expiration date. You'll also see chickens labeled *free range, organic*, or *natural*, but this doesn't mean much of anything. There's no guarantee that the chicken was not raised in a similar fashion to factory-farmed chickens. If it is labeled *organic*, it will not have been raised using antibiotics or chemicals but still might have been raised in a factory-type setting; if it says *natural* or *free range*, it may have been raised using antibiotics or chemicals, so you do need to check the package. I generally choose organic, free-range poultry.

Once thawed, it's important to use chicken sooner rather than later. One good strategy is to purchase chicken breasts or other parts in larger packs, use what you need, immediately divide the rest into single servings and place in zippered plastic bags, and freeze for later use. If you transfer them to the fridge the morning you want to use them, they'll be thawed by the time you get home.

Most of my recipes use boneless, skinless chicken breasts and thighs because they are readily available and easily stored and used. This is also the leaner choice, as they're lower in saturated fat than those with the skin on. Chicken thighs give recipes an especially rich flavor that chicken breasts cannot. Using rotisserie chickens from the grocery can offer a quick alternative to cooking a whole chicken yourself. Fusilli with Smoked Gouda and Chicken in (Chapter 7) uses rotisserie chicken as the main ingredient.

Most of us only think about eating turkey at the holidays. Now that so many turkey cuts are widely available, it can be a great meat choice for everyday. (See Chapter 7 for turkey breast; there are turkey burger recipes at DrGourmet.com/recipes.) Be cautious with ground turkey, though; often it is higher in fat and calories than ground beef is! Even worse, there's often added salt, with as much as 300 mg in a 4-ounce serving.

Beef

When I talk with patients about making changes for their health, they often say, "I'll just quit eating red meat"—and of course, never do. But occasionally eating red meat is okay for you. It is the choice of meat that is the most important factor. The rule of thumb is to not eat red meat more than about once per week and to focus on the percentage of fat in the meat you do eat.

Most people eat their beef in the form of ground beef. Look for the leanest you can find. One easy way to tell is "the redder, the better," because more fat in the ground beef will make it look pinker rather than darker red. You'll easily find ground beef labeled *80% lean* or *90% lean*. Subtract the number from 100 for the fat content (10% fat, for 90% lean ground beef, is better than 20% fat in the 80% beef). Your best choices are the even leaner—95% lean—which may be labeled *extra lean.*

The most tender and most expensive cuts of beef come from the tenderloin and include **tournedos** (medallions), which are from the smaller end, and the center-cut **filet mignon. Chateaubriand** comes from the larger end and is usually roasted. Most tenderloin recipes call for filet mignon.

Sirloin steaks are cut from just above or below the tenderloin. These can be a tasty and healthy cut and much less expensive. The steaks are more marbled and will be higher in fat, but even so there are only about 4 to 5 grams of fat in a 4-ounce serving. Top sirloin is more tender than bottom sirloin.

Round comes from the hip, and you'll find both top round and bottom round. As with sirloin, top round is more tender than bottom round. Round steaks can have as many as 9 to 10 grams of fat in a 4-ounce portion. Top round is often labeled *London broil,* although traditional London broil recipes actually use flank steak. Top round will work for London broil, however, and is economical, but I especially like using top round for stews.

Flank steak is perhaps my favorite cut of beef. It's lean, with only about 6 grams of fat in a 4-ounce serving, although it's less tender than some cuts because it comes from a muscle that gets used quite a bit. Try marinating your flank steak and cook it quickly over high heat. Like top and bottom round, flank steak can also be a good choice for stews. Similar to flank steak, **skirt steak** makes great steaks. It's cut from the same area as flank steak but is more marbled with fat than flank steak is.

Liver

Liver is an acquired taste for most people (not very many, I think), but it's really good for you. There is some confusion about whether liver is healthy for you, because liver does contain a lot of cholesterol (374 mg in a 4-ounce serving). There is also a misconception that liver is full of toxins.

The liver does make various enzymes that help the body eliminate toxins but those chemicals don't actually "build up" in the liver. It is very low in fat, however, with 5 grams of fat and 2 grams of saturated fat in 4 ounces. It is so good for you, with lots of vitamins, that there's general agreement that having it once a month or so is fine. Choose **calves' liver**, as it is less strongly flavored than beef liver and will be more tender.

Pork

Probably the most popular cut of pork are **pork chops.** Your best choices are center-cut boneless loin chops. Well trimmed, these are low in fat and calories, coming in at between 3 and 5 grams of fat per serving. **Pork loin** makes great roasts and is also low in fat and calories when trimmed carefully.

Another favorite cut is the juicy and succulent **tenderloin.** There are so many recipes that you can use pork tenderloin for—it's perfect for a dinner party, a weeknight family dinner, or a weekend barbecue.

Lamb

Lamb is pretty expensive, so I don't cook it very often. **Lamb shoulder** is more economical and is lean and flavorful. It can be harder to find, but it's worth it. The shoulder is leaner and has all the great lamb flavor, with only 148 calories in a 4-ounce serving (6 grams of fat and 2 grams of saturated fat). It can be used in almost any recipe that calls for a beef steak, and like beef, also can be cubed for kebabs and stews.

By far the most popular cut of lamb is **lamb chops.** They are higher in fat, but when trimmed to ⅛-inch fat, 4 ounces of lamb chops have 383 calories and 34 grams of fat (15 grams of saturated fat). Splurge on these at your favorite restaurant.

DAY 30 | DINNER

LEFTOVER BEEF STROGANOFF WITH EGG NOODLES (PAGE 180)

Day 30 Alternative Dinner Choices

Michael Angelo's Italian Natural Cuisine Lasagna with Meat Sauce

RESTAURANT MEALS

Ruby Tuesday Petite Sirloin

DAY 31 | HOW TO MAKE DINNER WHEN YOU'RE BUSY

Patients will often complain to me that they don't have time to cook. We are all busy these days, and you've read about how important I believe planning is for your health. Even so, our time is at a premium and there are times when you really are too busy to spend much time shopping and cooking.

Planning for those nights when you are busy is easy. The recipe for today is the perfect example of what I call a Pantry Meal™. Every one of these ingredients is easy to keep on hand and the whole recipe takes about 20 minutes' prep time (sometimes a bit longer to cook). The next time you are at the grocery store, buy these ingredients so you have them in your pantry, and you'll always have something quick and easy to make for dinner. You'll find other Dr. Gourmet Pantry Meals recipes online at Dr Gourmet.com/recipes/pantrymeals.

Having ingredients on hand is not just restricted to the pantry. Get your fridge and freezer into the act as well. Keeping a supply of frozen veggies lets you combine ingredients for everything from broccoli and cheese soup or cauliflower soup to almost any quick stir-fry. Don't limit yourself. Try onions, broccoli, carrots, cauliflower, edamame (shelled soybeans), green beans, and yellow corn. These frozen veggies, combined with a few other simple ingredients from the pantry, can make for many a great meal.

As you might have guessed by now, I always have a quality Parmigiano-Reggiano in my fridge. With a good Parmesan, you can use other standard ingredients, such as eggs and milk, to make almost anything—a frittata, scrambled eggs, macaroni and cheese, Parmesan salad dressing . . .

Crispy corn tortillas keep really well, and with a few ingredients you can make any number of tacos, a taco salad, or even a tamale pie.

Here's a list of some ideas to keep on hand:

Pantry:
Brown rice
Cornmeal (polenta)
Grits
Lentils
Quinoa
Taco shells
Whole wheat pasta

Canned or in cartons:
No-salt-added black beans
No-salt-added garbanzos (chickpeas)
No-salt-added pinto beans
No-salt-added white beans
No-salt-added chicken stock
Low-sodium cream of mushroom soup
Diced tomatoes

Frozen:
Broccoli
Cauliflower
Carrots
Edamame
Green beans
Lean ground beef
Onions
Peas
Yellow corn

Shrimp Enchiladas

SERVINGS: 4 ▎ **SERVING SIZE:** 3 ENCHILADAS ▎ THIS RECIPE CAN EASILY BE MULTIPLIED
▎ **COOKING TIME:** 30 MINUTES ▎ THE RECIPE MAKES GOOD LEFTOVERS. REHEAT GENTLY.

1 teaspoon olive oil
¼ cup dried pumpkin seeds
1 small onion, diced
1 red bell pepper, seeded
and diced
1 pound shrimp, peeled,
deveined, and coarsely
chopped
¼ teaspoon salt
½ teaspoon ground cumin
½ teaspoon paprika
½ teaspoon chili powder
12 (6-inch) corn tortillas
4 ounces Monterey Jack
cheese, grated

NUTRITION FACTS

Serving size 3 enchiladas
Servings 4
Calories 453
Calories from Fat 135
Total Fat 15 g (24%)
Saturated Fat 6 g (28%)
Trans Fat 0 g
Monounsaturated Fat 5 g
Cholesterol 188 mg (63%)
Sodium 510 mg (21%)
Total Carbohydrates 42 g (14%)
Dietary Fiber 7 g (27%)
Sugars 4 g
Protein 38 g
Vitamin A (32%)
Vitamin C (78%)
Calcium (34%)
Iron (31%)

*Parenthetical percentages
refer to % Daily Value.

This recipe was designed using frozen shrimp with frozen chopped onions and peppers. They're widely available and keep well. It's an example of having ingredients on hand that keep well and can be made into a meal within about 30 minutes.

1. Preheat the oven to broil. Place the olive oil in a large skillet over medium heat. Add the pumpkin seeds and cook for about 2 minutes, stirring frequently.

2. Add the onion and red bell pepper. Cook for about 2 minutes. Add the shrimp, salt, cumin, paprika, chili powder, and ½ cup of water. Cook, tossing frequently, for 8 to 10 minutes.

3. Divide the shrimp filling among the tortillas. Fold the tortillas as you fill them and place them on ovenproof plates (three to a plate). Top with 1 ounce of cheese for each plate, then place the plates under the boiler for about 1 minute until the cheese is melted. Serve.

Chef Tim Says . . . Eat Shrimp

There are two main types of shrimp: cold water shrimp and warm water shrimp. For the most part, the domestic shrimp available in U.S. markets is of the warm water variety and is caught in the Gulf of Mexico (think Bubba Gump Shrimp Company here). Thailand and South America, however, have become major exporters of shrimp to the world.

There are three common species of shrimp: white, pink. and brown.

Brown shrimp have a stronger flavor because of a higher iodine content. I have actually purchased brown shrimp that I couldn't eat because of the strong iodine flavor (this is rare).

White shrimp have shells that are a gray-green color. White shrimp are more delicate in flavor and generally cost more because of it, but they are your best choice. The Mexican white shrimp are very good, but most white shrimp on the market are farm raised in China.

Pink shrimp range in color from pink to a light yellow. The most common shrimp in markets today is known as Black Tiger shrimp. These guys are mostly farmed in Asia and are not of very consistent quality.

I used to vacation a lot along the coast of South Carolina and would go to the docks for fresh shrimp. The flavor is incomparable. Practically speaking, it's hard to buy fresh shrimp today because it's not widely available; most of the shrimp sold is processed and frozen quickly after catching. Because shrimp is so delicate, only the most careful handling will result in truly fresh product. Occasionally your local fish market may have fresh shrimp, but try to use it the day you buy it.

If it is handled well, shrimp that has been frozen and thawed is usually of very good quality. Look for firm shrimp with little softening of the shells. If the tail pulls away easily, it is not fresh. Quality shrimp, whether it is fresh or has been frozen, will have a fresh, clean odor. It should have the light salty smell of the ocean. Shrimp with dark spots (called *melanosis*) are not as fresh.

Day 31 Alternative Dinner Choices

CONVENIENCE MEALS

Lean Cuisine Szechuan Style Stir Fry with Shrimp

RESTAURANT MEALS

Baja Fresh Shrimp Ensalada

DAY 32 | DRINK ALCOHOL IF YOU LIKE, BUT ONLY IN MODERATION

I get questions from patients almost every day about whether it's safe or healthy for them to drink alcohol. It goes without saying that drinking too much alcohol is bad for you, but the best research we have now shows that those who consume two to three drinks per day for men or one to two per day for women live longer and healthier lives.

Moderation is the key to drinking alcohol healthfully.

The earliest meaningful research was done by a cardiologist named Arthur Klatsky. He noticed that many of his patients with heart disease weren't drinkers and this led him to do a retrospective study of over eighty thousand patients. He discovered that those who drank more had a much lower risk of dying from a heart attack. This research has since been repeatedly confirmed. One early study of Mediterranean countries showed the lowest risks of death from heart disease in those consuming the most alcohol. The important point, however, is that research on the Mediterranean diet shows that alcohol is generally consumed with meals.[7]

Women who drink red wine at least once per week are 16 percent less likely to get diabetes than are those women who don't drink regularly. Other alcoholic drinks, such as beer and spirits, yield similar results.[8]

It may be the antioxidants in wine that offer benefits beyond those of just grapes or grape juice. One study had a group drink 400 ml of wine each day while avoiding grapes and grape products.[9] The other group avoided alcohol of all kinds, as well as grapes and grape products, for two weeks. For the following two weeks, all of the volunteers returned to their normal diet in what is known as a "washout period," then for the next two weeks, the groups switched. Blood tests showed that those who drank the red wine each day had higher levels of antioxidants in their bloodstream and decreased levels of a substance used to measure the damage to cells. In theory, older volunteers would see greater benefits from the antioxidants in red wine, but that was not the case. The positive effects of drinking red wine was about the same regardless of age.

It does appear that wine may be the healthier choice over beer or spirits. Researchers in Spain recruited twenty healthy men between the ages of twenty-five and fifty to participate in a crossover study comparing cava (a sparkling wine containing a medium level of polyphenols) to gin (which has practically no polyphenols).[10] Each man consumed a specified amount of wine daily for a month, then switched to gin for a month, with a two-week period of abstaining from alcohol before and after each month of alcohol consumption. The subjects were directed to refrain from eating foods with high levels of polyphenols (such as onions, olive oil, and teas) but were given an otherwise Mediterranean-style diet designed to maintain their weight throughout the study.

The scientists performed blood tests on the subjects at the beginning and end of each period of alcohol consumption and found that although both gin and sparkling wine helped reduce the biomarkers of inflammation that indicate artherosclerosis, the effects of cava consumption were significantly better than were those seen for gin.

Even though cava is a white wine, the speculation is that the antioxidants in wine, especially red wine, offer protection from heart disease. Research on the substance resveratrol has grown out of this. In spite of some believing that this antioxidant is the miracle cure for everything, we don't really know exactly why drinking red wine or alcohol reduces the risk of heart disease. It may be that moderate daily consumption increases HDL cholesterol and reduces LDL cholesterol. It's clear that this isn't true of binge drinking, though. Saving up those two drinks a day and having fourteen on the weekend has been shown to be more harmful than not drinking at all.

What counts as a "drink?" That depends on what you are drinking. Most research uses the measure of a drink as 5 ounces of wine, 12 ounces of beer, or 1½ ounces of liquor. Remember that all alcohol, no matter how good for you, contains calories. There are about 125 calories in a 5-ounce glass of wine, 150 in a 12-ounce can of beer, and about 75 in an ounce of spirits such as whiskey or vodka.

I don't tell my patients who don't drink to start drinking. But for those who do drink, I caution them to imbibe in moderation and to do as folks who live around the Mediterranean do: Have a glass or two of wine with dinner.

DAY 32 | DINNER

PORTOBELLO BURGER AND SPICED SNAP PEAS

Dr. Tim Says . . .
IF THE LABEL SAYS . . .

Lean or extra lean: *Lean* means meat, poultry, or seafood cannot have more than 10 grams of fat in each 3-ounce serving. Lean foods must also have less than 4 grams of saturated fat and less than 95 milligrams of cholesterol per serving.

Extra lean means that the meat cannot have any more than 5 grams of fat in a 3-ounce serving. If a food is labeled *extra lean*, it can't have more than 2 grams of saturated fat and must contain less than 95 milligrams of cholesterol in each serving.

Light or lite: A food labeled *lite* or *light* means that it has one-third fewer less calories or half the amount of fat or sodium of the regular food.

Unfortunately, products that are light in color or texture may also be labeled *light*. A good example of this is light brown sugar. The manufacturer does have to tell you when the word *light* refers to color or texture.

Dr. Tim Says . . .
IF THE LABEL SAYS . . .

Fresh: The law doesn't mandate a definition for the term *fresh* but the FDA has created regulations that food manufacturers must follow, because the agency felt that this term was being misused on food labels.

The definition states that *fresh* can be placed on a label only "when it is used to suggest that a food is raw or unprocessed." This means that it can only be used when a food is raw, has not been frozen, has not been heated, and contains no preservatives.

Terms such as *fresh frozen, frozen fresh*, and *freshly frozen* are allowed if the food has been quickly frozen while fresh. If the food is blanched before freezing, the term *fresh* can still be used.

Natural: Watch out for this term. There is no guideline for what "natural" means. It could mean that the food has 50 percent lard or has a lot of sugar in it. The term *natural* has nothing to do with whether a food is healthy.

Healthy: For a food to be labeled *healthy*, it must be both low in fat and low in saturated fat. The product must also have no more cholesterol or sodium than recommended by the FDA. It does not mean the food is sugar free.

Some products use the word *healthy* in their brand name. The rule is that if the brand name was already in use when the law was passed in 1989, the company can continue using the name. Be careful, because this may not mean that the food is actually all that healthy. Turn the package over and check the Nutrition Facts.

Portobello Burger

SERVINGS: 1 ▌ **SERVING SIZE:** 1 BURGER ▌ THIS RECIPE CAN EASILY BE MULTIPLIED ▌
COOKING TIME: 30 MINUTES

Spray olive oil
1 (3-ounce) portobello
    mushroom cap
2 tablespoons barbecue
    sauce (low-sodium if
    possible)
1 ounce provolone cheese,
    sliced
2 slices tomato
2 slices onion
2 leaves lettuce
Freshly ground black
    pepper
1 whole wheat hamburger
    bun

NUTRITION FACTS

Serving size 1 burger
Servings 1
Calories 304
Calories from Fat 86
Total Fat 10 g (15%)
Saturated Fat 5 g (26%)
Trans Fat 0 g
Monounsaturated Fat 3 g
Cholesterol 19 mg (6%)
Sodium 507 mg (21%)
Total Carbohydrates 42 g (14%)
Dietary Fiber 5 g (20%)
Sugars 16 g
Protein 14 g
Vitamin A (15%)
Vitamin C (12%)
Calcium (29%)
Iron (10%)

*Parenthetical percentages
refer to % Daily Value.

Portobello mushrooms are actually large cremini mushrooms, and have become popular in the last few years because of their savory, meaty flavor. As mushrooms mature, the ring that protects the spores breaks and as a result there is loss of moisture. Young mushrooms contain as much as 80 percent water, and as they lose water (as portobellos do by having their gills exposed), the savory mushroom flavor is increasingly concentrated.

If you are going to use portobellos in a recipe that has liquid or a sauce, scraping the gills from the mushrooms before cooking will keep the sauce from turning black. Some flavor will be lost, but there will still be plenty of rich mushroom flavor.

1. Place a large ovenproof skillet in the oven and preheat the oven to 425°F.

2. When the oven is hot, spray the pan lightly with oil and place the mushroom in it gill side up. Spread the barbecue sauce over the gills of the mushroom. Bake for about 5 minutes and then turn over. Bake for another 5 minutes and turn one more time.

3. If you like your bun toasted, place it on the rack in the oven. After 2 minutes, remove the bun and place the mushroom on the bottom half. Top with the cheese, tomato, onion, lettuce, black pepper, and the top of the bun.

Spiced Snap Peas

SERVINGS: 2 ▌ SERVING SIZE: ABOUT 1 CUP ▌ THIS RECIPE CAN EASILY BE DOUBLED OR TRIPLED ▌ COOKING TIME: 15 MINUTES

2 teaspoons olive or grapeseed oil
1 tablespoon shallot, minced
8 ounces snap peas
⅛ teaspoon salt
¼ teaspoon ground nutmeg
¼ teaspoon ground ginger

NUTRITION FACTS

Serving size 1 cup
Servings 2
Calories 92
Calories from Fat 43
Total Fat 5 g (7%)
Saturated Fat 1 g (4%)
Trans Fat 0 g
Monounsaturated Fat 3 g
Cholesterol 0 mg (0%)
Sodium 151 mg (6%)
Total Carbohydrates 10 g (3%)
Dietary Fiber 3 g (12%)
Sugars 5 g
Protein 3 g
Vitamin A (26%)
Vitamin C (113%)
Calcium (5%)
Iron (14%)

*Parenthetical percentages refer to % Daily Value.

Peas are so good for you yet people often overlook snap peas or snow peas. This is a quick and easy recipe that takes only a few extra minutes for your weeknight meals and adds so much to dinner.

1. Place the oil in a medium skillet over medium heat. Add the shallots and cook gently, stirring frequently.

2. Add the snap peas, salt, nutmeg, and ginger to the pan and stir. Cover and cook for about 20 minutes, stirring about every 5 minutes.

CONVENIENCE MEALS

Michael Angelo's Italian Natural Cuisine Four Cheese Lasagna

RESTAURANT MEALS

P. F. Chang's Steamed Vegetable Dumplings

DAY 33 | WHAT ABOUT DESSERT?

I believe that part of the problem with obesity is that candy, desserts, sweets, and treats have become the norm and not the occasional dish they should be. Desserts are an important part of eating healthy, but they should be a special part of your life and not something for every day.

I have not included desserts in the menus, but you can find recipes for healthy desserts at DrGourmet.com/recipes/desserts. When you're working on losing weight, dessert should be a substitute for a meal portion about once a week. The goal for dessert recipes is less than 200 calories per serving, and it's a good goal for you to keep in mind when looking for desserts or dessert recipes.

One of the easiest, most refreshing and satisfying desserts is fresh fruit, and it's best to simply choose what is fresh and in season. Toss your fruit with about ½ teaspoon of sugar per serving and chill for an hour, and you'll have a sweet syrup. Top that with a spritz of canned whipped cream and you have the perfect healthy dessert at only about 125 calories.

You don't have to make your own dessert; it's a good idea to find some that you like to have around, so you can plan for your desserts just as you do your other meals. Frozen treats are good choices, and here are some that we've reviewed on the Dr. Gourmet Web site:

Breyer's No Sugar Added Ice Cream
Edy's Light No Sugar Added Ice Cream

Good Karma Organic Rice Divine Mint Chocolate Swirl
Healthy Choice No Sugar Added Ice Cream
Häagen-Dazs Fat Free Sorbets
Häagen-Dazs Raspberry & Vanilla Frozen Yogurt Bars
Häagen-Dazs Chocolate Sorbet Bar
Stonyfield Farm Organic Frozen Yogurt: Crème Caramel
Stonyfield Farm Organic Frozen Yogurt: Gotta Have Java
Stonyfield Farm Organic Frozen Yogurt: Low-Fat Minty Chocolate
    Chip
Stonyfield Farm Organic Frozen Yogurt: Vanilla Fudge Swirl
Turkey Hill No Sugar Added Ice Cream
Turtle Mountain Purely Decadent Dairy Free Mint Chocolate
    Chip
Weight Watchers Smart Ones Chocolate Éclair

For those with less willpower, a good strategy can be to buy desserts that come in individual packs like these:

Nabisco 100 Calorie Packs Chips Ahoy Thin Crisps
Nabisco 100 Calorie Packs Planters Peanut Butter Cookie Crisps

Likewise, if you can't keep sweets in the house without eating them, that's okay—just don't keep them in the house. Make plans to go out and have a (small) treat at the frozen yogurt store.

No matter what you choose, eat your dessert, make sure it's one that you love, and enjoy it!

DAY 33 | DINNER

PAELLA AND CRÈME BRÛLÉE

Paella

SERVINGS: 4 ▍ **SERVING SIZE:** 1½ CUPS PAELLA ▍ THIS RECIPE CAN EASILY BE MULTIPLIED
▍ **COOKING TIME:** 45 MINUTES ▍ THESE KEEP WELL FOR ABOUT 48 HOURS IN THE FRIDGE

60 threads saffron
¼ cup boiling water
2 teaspoons olive oil
2 cloves garlic, minced
½ large white onion,
  chopped
1 cup arborio rice
1½ cups chicken stock
¼ teaspoon salt
3 ounces low-fat, low-sodium
  turkey or chicken
  sausage, cut into
  ¼-inch disks
½ red bell pepper, seeded
  and cut into ½-inch
  pieces
4 ounces boneless chicken
  breast, cubed
6 ounces shrimp, peeled
  and deveined
12 littleneck clams
1 cup frozen peas

NUTRITION FACTS

Serving size 1½ cups paella
Servings 4
Calories 396
Calories from Fat 47
Total Fat 5 g (8%)
Saturated Fat 1 g (5%)
Trans Fats 0 g
Monounsaturated Fat 2 g
Cholesterol 99 mg (33%)
Sodium 634 mg (26%)
Total Carbohydrates 55 g (18%)
Dietary Fiber 4 g (17%)
Sugars 5 g
Protein 30 g
Vitamin A (32%)
Vitamin C (73%)
Calcium (7%)
Iron (60%)

*Parenthetical percentages
refer to % Daily Value.

Spanish food is some of the healthiest in the world. Paella is a great way for you to experience the rich flavors of this fantastic cuisine: healthy proteins, veggies, and rice, all flavored with rich saffron. The best part: It takes only one pan for cooking.

1. Place the saffron threads in a small cup and pour the ¼ cup of boiling water over them. Let stand to steep while preparing the other ingredients.

2. Place the olive oil in a large nonstick skillet over medium heat. Add the garlic and cook slowly for about 5 minutes, until the garlic begins to soften. Add the onion and cook for another 5 minutes.

3. Add the rice and cook for about 2 minutes, until the onion and rice are well blended. Add the chicken stock, 2¼ cups of water, and the salt. Stir and increase the heat to medium-high. After the mixture comes to a boil, lower the heat so that the rice is simmering. Stir the rice occasionally to keep it from sticking to the pan.

4. After about half of the liquid has cooked away in the rice, add the sausage.

5. When the rice is almost done (it should feel slightly grainy when tasted), add the red pepper and chicken and stir. Add up to ¼ cup of water, as needed. As the rice is just losing its graininess, add the shrimp, clams, and peas, and stir. Serve hot.

Dr. Tim Says . . . Look for Low-Fat/Low-Sodium Sausages

There are sausages that are lower in fat and salt that taste great. Look for ones that have about 2.5 grams of fat and no more than about 250 mg sodium per ounce. If you can't find them, that's okay. You can purchase other sausages: just precook them and then set them on a paper towel to drain.

Chef Tim Says . . . Eat Saffron

Saffron filaments are the dried red pistils of crocus flowers. For me this has always been a lovely twist of fate, because crocuses are my favorite flower. I remember that they were the first flower that I could call by name, because our front yard was covered with them. Little did I know their value.

Describing the flavor of saffron is difficult because the taste is so complex. It is at once aromatic, woody, and umami, with just a touch of sweetness. To me, saffron tastes yellow—like a warm summer day in the woods.

I suppose that you could go out in the yard and pick the flowers, pulling the stigmas out for drying, but I prefer to pick up a few grams at the store. Besides, a gram of saffron is about five hundred threads. As each flower only yields three threads, going to the market is quite a bit easier. Most of the available saffron is harvested in Spain, but countries in the Middle East including Iran are popular producers. The latter saffron is not as intense to my palate and I generally try to find the Spanish import.

How much saffron to use? I generally use about ten threads per serving, counting them out carefully. For some recipes I will make a saffron infusion—essentially saffron tea. I place the saffron in the bottom of a Pyrex measuring cup and add about ¼ cup of boiling water. Letting the threads steep in this way results in a more powerfully aromatic saffron flavor, especially in quick-sauté recipes.

For you saffron junkies out there, John Humphries has written a lovely book called *The Saffron Companion*. I must admit that I don't purchase many specialty cookbooks like this, but his writing is so wonderful and because most of the recipes are Mediterranean or Middle Eastern, they are both delicious and healthy.

Crème Brûlée

SERVINGS: 4 ▌ SERVING SIZE: 1 CUSTARD ▌ THIS RECIPE CAN EASILY BE MULTIPLIED BY 2 ▌ COOKING TIME: 60 MINUTES ▌ THE CUSTARDS KEEP WELL FOR A FEW DAYS. WRAP TIGHTLY WITH PLASTIC WRAP.

2 cups 2% milk
½ cup nonfat dry milk powder
1 teaspoon pure vanilla extract
6 tablespoons granulated Splenda or stevia
2 large egg yolks
⅛ teaspoon salt
8 teaspoons granulated sugar

NUTRITION FACTS

Serving size 1 custard
Servings 4
Calories 161
Calories from Fat 42
Total Fat 5 g (7%)
Saturated Fat 2 g (12%)
Trans Fats 0 g
Monounsaturated Fat 1 g
Cholesterol 116 mg (39%)
Sodium 199 mg (8%)
Total Carbohydrates 20 g (7%)
Dietary Fiber 0 g (0%)
Sugars 19 g
Protein 9 g
Vitamin A (7%)
Vitamin C (3%)
Calcium (29%)
Iron (2%)

*Parenthetical percentages refer to % Daily Value.

This recipe has origins in Italian and Spanish custards. It's a lot easier to make than you thought and makes the perfect dessert.

1. Place the milk, milk powder, and vanilla in a medium-size nonreactive saucepan. Heat over medium heat until the mixture reaches 180°F. (This is the temperature at which the milk will just begin to boil and at a higher temperature it will boil over.) Stir continuously and do not allow to boil.

2. Remove from the heat and allow to cool for at least a few hours (preferably overnight in the refrigerator).

3. After the milk mixture is cool, preheat the oven to 300°F. Fill a roasting pan with water to a level that will be about three-quarters of the way up the sides of a 1-cup ramekin. It is best to test this by placing the ramekins in the water bath to make sure the pan is not overfilled.

4. Place the roasting pan in the oven until the water is hot (this should take at least 20 minutes).

5. In a stainless-steel bowl, combine the Splenda, egg yolks, and salt. Cream together until smooth.

6. Strain the milk mixture through a fine sieve into the egg mixture. Whisk until well blended.

7. Divide the custard mixture among four 1-cup ramekins. Place the ramekins carefully in the hot water bath, return the roasting pan to the oven, and bake for 1 hour.

8. Very carefully remove the roasting pan from the oven and allow the custard to cool for 30 minutes while still in the water bath. Cover each custard with plastic wrap and chill overnight.

9. Place 2 teaspoons of sugar on the top of each custard. Using a blowtorch, melt the sugar by carefully aiming the tip of the flame at the surface of the sugar. Tilt and rotate the ramekin so that the melted sugar covers the surface of the custard.

Alternatively, the sugar can be melted under a broiler, but the custard will need to cool again afterward for about 10 minutes on the counter and for another 20 minutes in the refrigerator.

Day 33 Alternative Dinner Choices

CONVENIENCE MEALS

Kashi Southwest Style Chicken

RESTAURANT MEALS

Baja Fresh "Baja-Style" Tacos with Chicken

Dr. Tim Says . . .
IF THE LABEL SAYS . . .

Reduced, reduced fat, reduced calorie, reduced cholesterol, or reduced sodium: When you see the word *reduced*, it means that the food has to have at least 25 percent less fat, calories, cholesterol, or sodium than the regular food. For instance, reduced-fat mayonnaise has to have 25 percent less fat than regular mayonnaise does. This doesn't always mean that there will be *fewer calories*.

Some cookies are labeled *low fat*, but they actually have as many or more calories because the manufacturer put in more sugar, flour, or another high-calorie ingredient to help improve the flavor of the cookie. Check the label carefully. If the label uses the word *less* or *fewer*, it has the same meaning as reduced (less calories = reduced calories = fewer calories).

Percent fat free, or % fat free: If you see a label with the claim that the product is a certain percent fat free (e.g., "99% fat free"), it has to be a low-fat food. By definition, this means that it must have 3 grams of fat or less per serving.

There's good research about snacking. It seems most of us are one of two types. We are either sweet snackers or salty/savory snackers. Knowing which you are can help you manage your weight by making sure you have snacks on hand that will be satisfying. This doesn't mean that you need to schedule every one of your snacks, but having the right snack available will help you keep from eating things you should avoid.

Research shows that those who are fruit lovers eat sweet snacks more often and those who are veggie lovers will choose salty or savory snacks.[11] Knowing this about yourself helps you choose healthier options so you can keep your cupboard full of better choices.

I am certainly not a fan of snack foods, but if you are going to choose processed snacks, there's good research to show that air can help you eat less. One example is the dense, crispy Cheetos vs. the puffed version.[12] You'll eat fewer calories if you choose puffed snacks that take up a lot of volume and are less calorie dense. Popcorn is another good example of this. It makes a great snack and you'll find 100-calorie bags of microwave popcorn at the grocery store. These are filling, satisfying, have a lot of fiber, and should be in every salty snacker's pantry.

Nuts are your best choice if you are a salty/savory snacker. They're filling, stay with you, and are full of great monounsaturated fats. Eating nuts instead of carbohydrate-heavy snacks such as corn chips doesn't result in weight gain, and this is true even when folks eat more calories by eating nuts. We also know that eating nuts can help improve cholesterol profiles. Keep almonds, peanuts, walnuts, pecans, and other nuts on hand for your snacks.

What about sweet snackers? People try to tell me that their weight problems are the result of eating chocolate. When I discuss this with them, it's clear that the chocolate they are eating is not very satisfying and they are eating it impulsively. The secret to eating your chocolate and not gaining weight is to keep small portions of really great-quality chocolate in your cupboard. Make it a treat, not an everyday occurrence, and when you do eat it, take your time and enjoy it! We also know that sweet snackers are just as satisfied eating fruit as they are chocolate.

In one study, women were asked to eat an apple, a piece of chocolate, or nothing. They were given random instructions about when to eat their snack and then asked to record their mood afterward. Their mood in the 30 minutes after their snack was essentially the same, no matter what they ate. They were equally satisfied with the apple as with the chocolate (though chocolate did have a slight edge). The moods they recorded were much different, however, over time. After 90 minutes, the women felt much guiltier for eating the chocolate than the apple. Interestingly, the apple resulted in the same mood as did eating nothing (which is to say, no feelings of guilt).[13]

If you are a sweet snacker, keep your fridge full of fruit: apples, oranges, pears, grapes. Dried fruit is a great choice as well, and having raisins, apricots, and so on in your cupboard makes sense. Other great choices are low-calorie yogurt, pudding, Jell-O, Popsicles, and Fudgesicles.

Snacking is important. You need to have something when you're hungry and having the right snack on hand makes this easy for you.

Baked Ziti

SERVINGS: 6 ▌ **SERVING SIZE:** 2.67 OUNCES PASTA ▌ IF MULTIPLYING THIS RECIPE, USE MORE THAN ONE BAKING PAN ▌ **COOKING TIME:** 60 MINUTES ▌ LEFTOVERS ARE GREAT! THEY CAN BE DIVIDED AND PLACED IN ZIPPERED PLASTIC BAGS AND FROZEN. SAVE LEFTOVERS FOR DAY 36.

1 medium-size yellow pepper, peeled, seeded, and cut into 1-inch squares
1 medium-size red pepper, peeled, seeded, and cut into 1-inch squares
½ pound cremini mushrooms, halved
1 cup small shallots, peeled
Spray olive oil
1 pound whole wheat ziti
3 cups tomato sauce
1 tablespoon fresh rosemary
1 tablespoon fresh thyme
3 ounces fontina cheese, shredded
Freshly ground black pepper
1 ounce Parmigiano-Reggiano, grated

NUTRITION FACTS

Serving size ⅙ casserole (2.67 ounces of pasta)
Servings 6
Calories 444
Calories from Fat 76
Total Fat 9 g (13%)
Saturated Fat 4 g (20%)
Trans Fat 0 g
Monounsaturated Fat 3 g
Cholesterol 21 mg (7%)
Sodium 271 mg (11%)
Total Carbohydrates 74 g (25%)
Dietary Fiber 5 g (21%)
Sugars 8 g
Protein 19 g
Vitamin A (31%)
Vitamin C (224%)
Calcium (22%)
Iron (24%)

*Parenthetical percentages refer to % Daily Value.

Baked pasta dishes are perfect for your healthy diet. Use lots of roasted veggies for savory flavor, add high-fiber whole wheat pasta, and top with rich cheese.

1. Preheat the oven to 375°F.

2. Place the peppers, mushrooms, and shallots in a roasting pan and spray lightly with olive oil.

3. Place the roasting pan in the preheated oven and roast the vegetables until slightly soft, 15 to 20 minutes.

4. While the vegetables are roasting, bring 5 quarts of water to a boil and add the ziti. Cook until slightly underdone, 12 to 15 minutes. Drain.

5. Prepare a 12 by 9 by 2-inch oblong pan (Pyrex is a good choice) by lightly spraying the inside with olive oil. Set aside. (Lining the pan with nonstick aluminum foil works as well.)

6. Place the tomato sauce, rosemary, thyme, fontina cheese, and black pepper in a glass or stainless-steel bowl. Stir well and add the ziti. Toss the pasta to coat well.

7. Add the vegetables and gently fold together until well blended. Pour the ingredients into the prepared pan.

8. Sprinkle the grated cheese over the top.

9. Bake at 375°F for 15 to 20 minutes, until the top is slightly browned.

Chef Tim Says . . . Eat Mushrooms

White Mushrooms: White (button) mushrooms are the most common of the thousands of varieties of mushrooms and the most readily available in markets today. They vary in size, but mushroom growers use the term *white mushroom* to refer to those that are over an inch in diameter. Many recipes use the term *button mushroom*, referring to smaller cultivated white mushrooms.

Freshness is easy to spot with white mushrooms. Avoid those with dark spots or that are soft, squishy, or whose surface feels slimy. Turn the mushroom over and check to see if the gills are exposed. This is the best indicator of freshness. The ring is the soft covering that joins the edge of the cap to the stem, and if it is not intact and the gills can be seen, the mushroom is past its prime.

The idea of not rinsing mushrooms because they absorb water is myth. Mushrooms are about 80 percent water to start with and numerous published tests have not shown that there is a significant amount of water absorbed when mushrooms are washed.

Cremini: Cremini mushrooms are marketed under many names, including baby bella, Roman, Italian, brown, or classic brown mushrooms. They are similar in size to white mushrooms but are a light cocoa color and have a firmer texture. They are much more flavorful than white mushrooms, having a richer, earthy taste that activates the umami taste buds. Their flavor has often been referred to as "meaty."

Dr. Tim Says . . .

IF THE LABEL SAYS . . .

Low: The word *low* has very specific meanings.

Low calorie means 40 calories or less per serving.

Low cholesterol means 20 milligrams or less cholesterol per serving.

Low fat means 3 gram of fat or less per serving.

If a package claims that the food is *low in saturated fat*, it has to have 1 gram or less saturated fat in each serving.

Low sodium means 140 milligrams or less sodium per serving.

Very low sodium means 35 milligrams or less sodium per serving.

The words *low source of, few, little,* or *small amounts of* mean the same thing as *low*. For instance, low calorie = few calories = low source of calories.

Unsalted or no sodium/salt added: *Unsalted* or *no sodium/salt added* means that there has not been any salt added to the food. Keep in mind that this doesn't mean that the food will actually be low in sodium. Some foods that contain ingredients naturally high in sodium, such as baking soda, miso, flour, celery, and crab, could technically be labeled *no sodium/salt added*.

CONVENIENCE MEALS

Healthy Choice Naturals Pumpkin Squash Ravioli

RESTAURANT MEALS

Panera Half-Serving Mediterranean Veggie Sandwich with a Fruit Cup

DAY 35 | *YOUR KEY TO EATING HEALTHY IS UNDERSTANDING TASTE*

I have spent years working to convince folks that eating healthy and eating great foods are the same thing. Most folks believe that if a dish is healthy, it just can't taste good. This is simply not true. Research supports: Being told a dish is "healthy," people feel it will not taste good—yet in blind taste tests, they will more often choose the healthier version as their favorite.

So how do you create or recognize recipes that you'll love to eat over and over? Understanding the flavors in foods can help you understand your own preferences.

Our tongues have five types of receptors that sense flavors: salt, sweet, bitter, sour, and one called umami. Contrary to what you might have read or heard elsewhere, there is no "taste map" of the tongue. We now know that taste buds are not localized to certain areas of the tongue but are in fact distributed more evenly. We know that each type of taste bud acts on its own, but the way they interact with one another is just as important. We also know that stimulating any one taste bud enhances others. Knowing how taste works and how the different tastes blend with one another is how you can get great results when you're cooking for yourself and can help you eat better.

Sweet

Most all of us love sweet tastes, and sweet flavors are more easily distinguished than other tastes. As strong as our sweet taste buds are, they are just as important because of the way they enhance other flavors. You may love bitter flavors, but for most of us those bitter tastes are far better for some sweetness. Lemonade is the perfect example of this.

Salty

It takes very little salt to stimulate the salt taste receptors, so it takes very little salty flavor to help enhance and complement other taste buds. That's why it's crucial for you to add salt to most dishes to help with the balance of flavors. For instance, a little sodium in sweet dishes will enhance the sugary flavor: Almost all chocolate contains just a little salt.

It's important that you understand that it's okay to use salt in your recipes. As I have mentioned before, measuring is the important rule. Over time, I have come to find that it takes about 300 to 400 milligrams of sodium per serving (about ⅛ teaspoon) in a dish to adequately stimulate the salt taste buds.

Salty flavors react with acidic foods to soften the sour flavors.

Sour

Your sour taste buds are stimulated by acidic foods, such as citrus fruits, and they react very quickly. These flavors will often present themselves early and then be softened by salty and sweet tastes. Used carefully, they can brighten almost any dish—but they can also easily overpower a recipe.

Bitter

Bitter and sour are not the same. Examples of bitter tastes include such things as cabbage, spinach, and collard or mustard greens. My Collard Greens recipe (page 41) provides one of the best examples of how to balance flavors. I combine the bitter collard greens with a little maple syrup, salt, and lemon to hit four flavor notes for a nearly perfect recipe.

Umami

Umami has become one of my favorite words. I just love saying it. Umami, umami, umami . . .

This taste was first identified by Professor Kikunae Ikeda in the early 1900s. He felt that the recognized tastes—sweet, salty, sour, and bitter—could not fully explain the rich flavors of such foods as cheese, mushrooms, and meat. He began experimenting with a broth of the seaweed *konbu*, which is a staple of the Japanese diet.

The professor felt that *konbu* contained the unique savory flavor that is distinct from the traditional four tastes. He found that glutamate crystals extracted from the seaweed reproduced the same flavor sensation as savory foods. One of the first uses of this new information was unfortunately the creation of monosodium glutamate (MSG). MSG has since been used as a flavor enhancer in foods. It is an obstacle to eating healthy because of the large amount of sodium that it adds to foods. (It also appears that it may stimulate weight gain!)[14] We now know that chemicals other than glutamate, such as inosinate and guanylate, also activate the umami taste buds.

For years, the feeling of Western researchers was that there were only four proven taste buds and that all flavors were felt to be the sensation of one or more of them being stimulated. Savory flavors were explained away as a complex combination of two or more of the taste buds being activated. As with many things scientific, "proof" can be a moving target, and umami taste buds have now been "discovered" by the West.

At some point in my restaurant career, a chef told me that the definition of *gourmet* was when all of the flavors of the ingredients in a particular dish were easily distinguished. So for the perfect tomato sauce you should be able to taste each ingredient: garlic, onions, olive oil, basil, tomatoes, salt, pepper, and so on.

I work to create recipes based on this ideal, and knowing about the fifth, umami, taste makes creating healthy recipes so much easier. It is the *balance* of flavors, not one individual ingredient, which makes a dish. When a dish is just salty enough with an umami undertone and a touch of sweetness, all balancing sour or bitter flavors, you're more likely to enjoy it (and it doesn't matter that it's "healthy").

We also react to umami tastes in a way that is very comforting (think mac and cheese), and emphasizing those flavors in your recipes will help you be more satisfied. As you are looking for recipes to try, think about the umami flavors in the dish. How can they be enhanced? For instance, sweating mushrooms until they are caramelized intensifies their rich umami flavor. The best-quality Parmesan and aged cheeses have a more intense umami flavor, so you can use less in your recipes. A single ounce of Parmigiano-Reggiano adds a complex, mellow flavor to a recipe.

Here are some other common umami foods that you can use as a guide when looking for recipes:

- Mushrooms
- Dried porcini mushrooms (Ground into a powder, it is essentially pure umami powder and will enhance almost any recipe, with no added calories.)
- Truffles
- Beef
- Pork
- Lamb
- Cheese, with aged cheeses being more savory
    Parmigiano-Reggiano
    Pecorino Romano
- Eggs
- Garlic (especially roasted garlic)
- Roasted nuts
- Soy sauce (Even though soy sauce has lots of sodium, it can be a great savory ingredient.)
- Clams

- Oysters
- Shrimp
- Tuna
- Tomatoes
- Caramelizing foods such as onions enhances the umami flavor

The best chefs know these principles and work hard to create dishes that touch on all five flavors. The same holds true for food manufacturers. Highly processed foods are finely tuned to balance tastes and create products that you will love. One problem is that they will often overuse sweet and salty flavors, leading to excess calories and sodium.

When you are looking at recipes, keep these five flavors in mind. The recipes that are going to be the most delicious and satisfying will have a balance of tastes. A foundation of umami ingredients with at least two other flavors—sweet and salty, or salty and sour, or sour and sweet—will make for the best meals. Ones that balance four or five tastes will have you feeling like you've been in a fine restaurant.

DAY 35 | DINNER

LEFTOVER PAELLA (PAGE 208)

Day 35 Alternative Dinner Choices

CONVENIENCE MEALS

Kashi Southwest Style Chicken

RESTAURANT MEALS

Baja Fresh Shrimp Ensalada

CHAPTER 6 | **WEEK 6 GOALS**

I have worked very hard to tell you what you can and should be eating. So many diet plans work by taking things away and that's tough, I think.

That said, there are some things you shouldn't do and some areas that can be a challenge. This week, I'll talk about the reasons you shouldn't eat fast food or drink soda. There's clear research showing just how bad both of these are for you. While I don't like convenience foods, there is a way to approach them so that you can make them work for you in getting and staying healthy.

Travel and dining out are part of your real world and have to be included in any plan. It's easy and there are two days devoted to finding and eating great food.

The end of your six-week plan closes out with a discussion of vitamins. Do you need supplements? After what you have learned in the first forty-one days, you'll see what works best.

This week, you'll:

▌ Learn why fast food really is bad for you (even the ones you thought might be healthy)
▌ Start eating out sensibly
▌ Understand what to drink

- Learn about how to incorporate convenience meals into your plan
- Learn why vitamin supplements don't work

WEEK 6 | MENU

A personalized shopping list for Week 6 can be found at DrGourmet .com/shoppinglist.

DAY 36 | DON'T EAT FAST FOOD

I have repeatedly laid responsibility for obesity in America squarely at the feet of the fast-food companies. A bit over the top, maybe, but I believe that this isn't too far-fetched. While there is no definitive study that says, "Fast food makes you fat," more than enough research proves it to be a major contributor to obesity.

The issue of increasing portion sizes is clearly at the top of the list of ways in which fast food contributes to obesity. In one study, a group of researchers at the University of Wisconsin estimated just how much supersizing costs you in the long run.[1] Their research took into account the difference in price between a regular and a supersized meal. At the same time, they estimated the weight gain over time from the added calories in the larger portions. Their bottom line? The larger meal cost an additional 17 percent at the cash register and provided an additional 73 percent more calories than did a regular meal. The hidden costs of the health problems from weight gain added somewhere between 123 and 191 percent to the overall cost of the meal. So supersize your meal and pay now, but pay even more later.

Such research and conclusions are supported by USDA estimates that put added health-care costs from obesity at $71 billion per year. If you haven't seen the film *Supersize Me*, do—this will show you just what happens

WEEK 6 MENU

RECIPE	CONVENIENCE FOOD ALTERNATIVE	RESTAURANT MEAL ALTERNATIVE
DAY 36		
Leftover Baked Ziti	Healthy Choice Naturals Pumpkin Squash Ravioli	Panera Half-Serving Mediterranean Veggie Sandwich with a Fruit Cup
DAY 37		
Red Beans and Rice	Michael Angelo's Signature Line Chicken Parmesan	Chili's Chicken Enchilada Soup
DAY 38		
Spaghetti and Meatballs and Salad with Parmesan Peppercorn Dressing	Lean Cuisine Spaghetti with Meat Sauce	Noodles and Company House Marinara (small) with Small Side Salad
DAY 39		
Sweet Red Pepper Barbecue Tuna, Cheesy Quinoa, and Roasted Cauliflower	Lean Cuisine Salmon with Basil	P. F. Chang's Oolong Marinated Sea Bass
DAY 40		
Leftover Spaghetti and Meatballs and Salad with Parmesan Peppercorn Dressing	Lean Cuisine Spaghetti with Meat Sauce	Noodles and Company House Marinara (small) with Small Side Salad
DAY 41		
Salmon with Caper Mayonnaise and Savory Quinoa	Lean Cuisine Salmon with Basil	Red Lobster Grilled Fish with Baked Potato and a Side Salad
DAY 42		
Pizza with Tomato, Basil, and Roasted Garlic	DiGiorno Rising Crust Three Mushroom Pizza	Pizza Hut Half-Serving Cheese Only Personal Pan Pizza

to your body when you eat fast food. In it, the documentarian Morgan Spurlock eats only at McDonald's for a month and supersizes the meals whenever offered the option at the cash register. The results documented in the film are devastating to his health. Although some of his symptoms could be attributed to melodrama, there's no refuting the change in his lab results, which show a marked increase in cholesterol and severe damage to his liver function.

So can it be done? Can you eat fast food and be healthy? Only if you're really, really careful. There are a number of people now who have eaten only at McDonald's but made more intelligent choices than in Mr. Spurlock's experiment and actually lost weight. After all, he did supersize most meals and often ate as many as 5,000 calories per day.

I have been in McDonald's for research to see what is available. Aesthetics aside, the food on offer is mostly hamburgers and these *are* inexpensive compared to the healthier options. Salads are five dollars (even though they likely cost less than their hamburgers to produce). Unfortunately not many more menu items could be considered healthy. The only inexpensive healthy options are such things as Chipotle BBQ Snack Wraps with Grilled Chicken. This is a reasonably healthy choice at only 260 calories and 8 grams of fat, but note that McDonald's calls this a *snack*. Their regular hamburger has 250 calories and 9 grams of fat, but it isn't labeled a snack. This sort of attitude doesn't lead to healthy eating—it leads to you to overeat.

Research shows that we're not very good at judging the number of calories we eat, especially in fast-food joints.[2] In one study, researchers approached diners in fast-food restaurants and asked them to self-report on their height and weight, and then to estimate the number of calories in the meal that they had just consumed. The interviewers had been watching and recording what the participants had eaten.

The interesting finding was that all of those interviewed underestimated the number of calories by an average of 23 percent. When the researchers looked at the estimates of larger meals vs. smaller ones, they found that when eating a smaller meal, people were able to more accurately estimate the number of calories they had eaten. This wasn't the case with larger meals, where the number of calories consumed was underestimated by a whopping 38 percent (or maybe I should say a Whopper).

The trick is for you to avoid as much as possible eating at fast-food joints. If you know you are going to, make sure that you know what you are going to eat *before* you set foot in the door. You can find a section on the Dr. Gourmet Web site with recommendations for the healthier choices from the major fast-food chains to help you plan.

DAY 36 | DINNER

LEFTOVER BAKED ZITI (PAGE 214)

Day 36 Alternative Dinner Choices

CONVENIENCE MEALS

Healthy Choice Naturals Pumpkin Squash Ravioli

RESTAURANT MEALS

Panera Half-Serving Mediterranean Veggie Sandwich with a Fruit Cup

DAY 37 | DRINK COFFEE OR TEA: THEY'RE GOOD FOR YOU

Coffee is another one of those things that patients will often tell me that they are going to stop consuming, when I speak with them about improving their health. I have yet to figure out how or why folks have come to believe that coffee is bad for you. There are, in fact, many studies showing that coffee is really good for you.

One outstanding study looked at the relationship between coffee and inflammatory conditions such as heart disease, cancer, Parkinson's disease, gallstones, cirrhosis of the liver, and diabetes.[3] The speculation is that antioxidants in coffee help to control inflammation in the same way as the antioxidants in vegetables, olive oil, and wine. Researchers looked at more than twenty-seven thousand postmenopausal women who did not have any inflammatory diseases.

After a period of fifteen years, the study showed that the more coffee a woman drank, the lower the death rates from these conditions. This was true even after controlling for age, smoking, and alcohol intake, even though women who drank more coffee tended to smoke and drink more alcohol.

In another large study, researchers in Italy[4] looked at over eleven thousand people who had already suffered a heart attack, to see if coffee increased the risk of a second heart attack or other cardiovascular problem. At the beginning of the study, and at regular intervals over the course of 3½ years, the subjects were questioned about diet—including their coffee intake. The diet and coffee consumption of those subjects who had a second heart attack or a stroke were compared with those subjects who had no further problems. It was clear that drinking coffee made no difference either way: participants didn't have a higher or lower risk of heart attack or stroke. (You have to love that the Italians did this study. They do know what is important in life!)

It appears that coffee might even help you keep from gaining weight. Research has shown that those increasing their coffee intake have a lower average weight gain over time. This certainly doesn't prove that coffee can help you lose weight, but men drinking an additional cup and a half of coffee per day gained only about a pound in one study. The same held true for women, and those whose BMI was over 25, those who smoked, or those who were less physically active seemed to gain even less weight after increasing their coffee intake.[5]

Patients will often claim that their blood pressure is higher because of drinking more coffee, but there's no solid evidence that drinking coffee will raise your blood pressure.

There is, however, some research that indicates it might help lower the risk of diabetes. In another study of more than twenty-eight thousand women aged fifty-five to sixty-nine, researchers assessed the impact of coffee on their risk of developing diabetes.[6] Those having more than six cups per day had a 34 percent lower risk! Drinking decaffeinated coffee showed an even greater effect, with a further reduction in the risk of diabetes by 42 percent.

This effect held true even though the women who drank more coffee also tended to drink more alcohol, smoke more, exercise less, and consume more high-fat dairy foods and less dietary fiber. Coffee is the single largest source of antioxidants in the Western diet and it's likely that this is what was offering them protection.

Tea is another good choice, especially iced tea as a replacement for soda. While it doesn't have the amount of antioxidants as coffee, it comes in at a close second when compared to any other food. For those of you who want to drink sweetened tea, I think that's fine. There are 9 teaspoons of sugar in a 12-ounce Coke. A teaspoon of sugar in iced tea is enough sweetness for almost everyone and adds only 16 calories (instead of the 140 in the soda). There is good research out of Japan on green tea and it's a great choice, too. The studies have been mixed but some small studies have shown easier weight loss occurs when two or three cups of green tea are consumed daily.

It's sort of like alcohol. If you don't like coffee or tea and are not drinking such beverages regularly, this doesn't mean you have to start. But if you are (like me) a fan of coffee, don't worry. It's good for you.

Red Beans and Rice

SERVINGS: 8 ▮ SERVING SIZE: ABOUT 1½ CUPS BEANS WITH ⅔ CUP RICE ▮ THIS RECIPE
CAN EASILY BE DOUBLED, BUT YOU'LL NEED A VERY LARGE POT ▮ COOKING TIME: 60
MINUTES ▮ THIS RECIPE TASTES EVEN BETTER AS LEFTOVERS. BEST TO MAKE IT ON SUN-
DAY FOR MONDAY AND LATER IN THE WEEK.

1 pound dried dark red
   kidney beans
1 teaspoon canola or
   grapeseed oil
1 large onion, diced
6 cloves garlic, minced
4 ribs celery, diced
1 large green bell pepper,
   seeded and diced
1 (14-ounce) package
   Healthy Choice or
   Healthy Ones smoked
   sausage, cut into
   ½ inch-disks
1 teaspoon dried thyme
3 teaspoons Chef Paul
   Prudhomme's Magic
   Salt Free or Salt-Free
   Tony Chachere's
   Creole Seasoning
1 teaspoon salt
Freshly ground black
   pepper
½ teaspoon Tabasco sauce
2 cups uncooked brown rice

Creating this recipe was a challenge, not so much because of the amount of fat that many Creole recipes have in them, but because of the typical amount of salt. The first concern was the sausage. A number of variations of ham and sausage were tried. Healthy Choice and Healthy Ones sausages are really tasty, with only 480 mg of sodium and 2.5 grams of fat in 2 ounces. You may be able to find similar products at your grocery—look for the American Heart Association heart-check symbol.

The other issue was the seasoning. There are countless recipes for Creole seasoning, but most of us don't have the time to make our own and will choose one off the shelf at the store. The ones made in Louisiana are the best: salt-free Chef Paul Prudhomme's and Tony Chachere's are great products! Aside from these, McCormick is the national brand with the lowest amount of sodium and it has terrific flavor, but if you use this one, don't add any salt.

Lastly, there is the issue of the beans. Most canned beans have a lot of salt in them, but you can use the low- or no-sodium versions in place of soaking and cooking dried beans. Rinse them well before adding them to the pot. Another great alternative is to use frozen kidney beans. I stumbled across a product by a company called Pictsweet and these work great. There's virtually no salt and the 32-ounce bag of frozen beans is about equivalent to a pound of dried beans.

Serving size about 1½ cups
beans with ⅔ cup rice
Servings 8
Calories 438
Calories from Fat 33
Total Fat 4 g (6%)
Saturated Fat 1 g (4%)
Trans Fat 0 g
Monounsaturated Fat 1 g
Cholesterol 10 mg (3%)
Sodium 443 mg (18%)
Total Carbohydrates 81 g (27%)
Dietary Fiber 18 g (70%)
Sugars 4 g
Protein 22 g
Vitamin A (8%)
Vitamin C (43%)
Calcium (12%)
Iron (38%)

*Parenthetical percentages
refer to % Daily Value.

1. Place the beans in a large bowl and cover with 3 quarts of water. Soak overnight, rinsing away the soaking water. (For a quicker way of preparing the dried beans, place the beans in a large stockpot and cover with 4 quarts of water. Bring the water to a boil, then lower the heat to medium-low heat and cook for about an hour while you are dicing the vegetables.)

2. Place the oil in a large stockpot over medium heat. Add the onion and garlic. Cook for about 5 minutes, stirring frequently. Add the celery and green pepper and cook, stirring frequently, for about 5 minutes.

3. Add the smoked sausage and cook for about 5 minutes, stirring frequently.

4. Drain the beans and add them to the pot, then add 8 cups water and the thyme, Creole seasoning, salt, ground pepper, and Tabasco sauce. Stir and lower the heat to medium-low. Cook for about 2 hours, stirring occasionally.

5. When the beans are done, place 6 cups water in a medium-size saucepan over high heat. When the water is boiling, add the rice, stir once, and lower the heat to medium-low. Cook until all the water is gone, about 25 minutes. Stir the rice once to fluff it and then serve the red beans over the rice in eight equal portions.

Day 37 Alternative Dinner Choices

CONVENIENCE MEALS

Michael Angelo's Signature Line Chicken Parmesan

RESTAURANT MEALS

Chili's Chicken Enchilada Soup

Drinking soda—even diet soda—is bad for you. It leads to obesity and subsequently to diabetes, high blood pressure, and heart disease. The soft drink industry would have you believe that drinking Coke or Pepsi isn't bad for your health, but their arguments are simply fantasy. It is clearly in their best interest to bend the truth so you feel good about drinking soda. They do, after all, get paid to sell you sugared water.

And that's not just a little bit of sugar but a whole lot. Remember: A single 12-ounce can of Coke has the equivalent of about 9 teaspoons of sugar. Nine teaspoons! That's why research has shown that having more than 2½ sugar-sweetened drinks per day significantly increases your risk of death from heart disease.

There is a huge body of research on soft drinks. One study showed that those who drink the most sugared soda have two-thirds higher risk of developing type 2 diabetes than those who don't drink soda. There's been controversy about whether sodas with high-fructose corn syrup might be worse for you. In this study, the researchers looked at the type of sugar consumed. Participants who consumed sodas with both fructose and glucose had an even higher risk of developing diabetes.[7]

Soda consumption is also linked with weight gain, and our kids are the most vulnerable. One study found that the more sweet drinks children consumed, the more quickly their body mass index rose as they grew. It didn't matter whether the drink was soda or a fruit juice: Both caused weight gain.[8] Additionally, our body doesn't process those calories in the same way as calories from whole foods. When you drink the 140 calories in a can of Coke, you aren't satisfied. The liquid doesn't fill you up in the same way that solid food does and the body stores those extra calories directly as fat.

Drinking diet soda has also been linked to obesity. The researchers of San Antonio Heart Study looked at soft drink consumption in a group of about 1,500 people they followed over eight years. When the study began, only 622 were normal weight. The study showed that the more soda participants consumed, the more likely they were to be overweight or obese at the end of the study. The interesting thing is that this was true for both sugared and sugar-free soft drinks. The researchers found that a single extra can of soda each day increased the risk of obesity by a whopping 41 percent. Those drinking more than two cans of diet soda per day were almost 60 percent more likely to be overweight![9]

Animal studies might offer some insight into why this is. It appears that the constant sweetness reduces one's natural ability to use sweet flavors to judge the caloric content of food. It is hard to draw perfect conclusions from animal studies, and drinking more sugar-free soda has not clearly been shown to impair the ability of humans to judge other food consumption. There is research, however, showing that those who drink more artificial sweeteners tend to gain more weight. While such studies don't prove that consuming diet drinks *causes* weight gain, it does clearly establish a link.

Drink water. Tea, green tea, and coffee are also well established to be good for you and are chock full of antioxidants. Make these a part of your life and skip the soda.

DAY 38 | DINNER

SPAGHETTI AND MEATBALLS AND SALAD WITH PARMESAN PEPPERCORN DRESSING

Spaghetti and Meatballs

SERVINGS: 1 ▮ **SERVING SIZE:** 6 MEATBALLS WITH 2 OUNCES PASTA AND ½ OUNCE CHEESE ▮ THIS RECIPE CAN EASILY BE MULTIPLIED. IF YOU ARE GOING TO MAKE MORE THAN TWO SERVINGS, ADD ABOUT A QUART OF BOILING WATER FOR EACH SERVING OF PASTA. ▮ **COOKING TIME:** 45 MINUTES

2 ounces spaghetti
4 meatballs (recipe follows)
½ cup tomato sauce
½ ounce Parmigiano-
    Reggiano, grated

NUTRITION FACTS

Serving size 6 meatballs,
    2 ounces pasta, ½ cup
    tomato sauce, ½ ounce
    Parmigiano-Reggiano
Servings 1
Calories 464
Calories from Fat 87
Total Fat 10 g (15%)
Saturated Fat 5 g (23%)
Trans Fat 0 g
Monounsaturated Fat 3 g
Cholesterol 59 mg (20%)
Sodium 548 mg (23%)
Total Carbohydrates 60 g (20%)
Dietary Fiber 4 g (17%)
Sugars 7 g
Protein 32 g
Vitamin A (10%)
Vitamin C (27%)
Calcium (22%)
Iron (32%)

*Parenthetical percentages
refer to % Daily Value.

You can use bottled tomato sauce for this recipe. I look for tomato sauce with 2 grams of fat or less per serving. Look carefully at the Nutrition Facts on the label, because some jars list the serving size as ¼ cup (not ½ cup, which is the standard serving). Look for ones that are lower in sugar as well.

1. Place 4 quarts of water in a medium-size to large stockpot (depending on the number of servings of pasta to be cooked) over high heat. When the water is boiling, add the spaghetti.

2. While the pasta is cooking, place the meatballs (recipe follows) and tomato sauce in a medium-size (or larger, if making multiple servings) saucepan and heat gently over medium heat. When the sauce is hot, lower the heat to low.

3. When the pasta is done, drain, then place in the sauce with the meatballs and toss well.

4. Serve hot in a large bowl, topped with the grated cheese.

Meatballs

SERVINGS: 4 ▊ **SERVING SIZE:** 6 MEATBALLS ▊ THIS RECIPE CAN EASILY BE DOUBLED OR TRIPLED ▊ **COOKING TIME:** 60 MINUTES ▊ THESE KEEP WELL FOR ABOUT 48 HOURS IN THE FRIDGE AFTER BEING COOKED. REHEAT GENTLY.

1 pound extra-lean ground beef (no more than 5% fat)
2 ounces fresh bread crumbs
1 teaspoon dried oregano
1 teaspoon dried basil
1 teaspoon dried rosemary
1 teaspoon dried thyme
½ teaspoon salt
⅛ teaspoon freshly ground black pepper
Spray olive oil

NUTRITION FACTS

Serving size 6 meatballs
Servings 4
Calories 219
Calories from Fat 63
Total Fat 7 g (11%)
Saturated Fat 3 g (14%)
Trans Fat 0 g
Monounsaturated Fat 3 g
Cholesterol 70 mg (23%)
Sodium 470 mg (20%)
Total Carbohydrates 11 g (4%)
Dietary Fiber 1 g (4%)
Sugars 1 g
Protein 26 g
Vitamin A (1%)
Vitamin C (1%)
Calcium (5%)
Iron (22%)

*Parenthetical percentages refer to % Daily Value.

This recipe is so versatile. You can use it for spaghetti and meatballs, meatball hoagies (use whole wheat rolls), or cut up on top of pizza. The key is to choose the leanest ground beef possible: look for 93% lean. You can always ask the butcher to grind some from a cut of bottom round. Make sure that the butcher trims away all of the excess fat before grinding.

1. Preheat the oven to 400°F. Place a large nonstick ovenproof skillet in the oven.

2. Mix the ground beef with the bread crumbs, herbs, salt, and pepper until well blended.

3. Roll the mixture into a large ball and cut in half. Roll each portion into two balls and cut each of those in half. Continue until there are twenty-four small meatballs. The meatballs are easy to form by rolling them in your palms until round and smooth.

4. Spray the hot skillet lightly with olive oil. Place the meatballs in the skillet and return the pan to the oven. Cook for 12 to 15 minutes, until they are firm to the touch.

Salad with Parmesan Peppercorn Dressing

SERVINGS: 8 ▌ **SERVING SIZE:** 2 TABLESPOONS ▌ THIS RECIPE CAN EASILY BE DOUBLED
OR TRIPLED ▌ **COOKING TIME:** 15 MINUTES ▌ THIS KEEPS WELL FOR ABOUT 4 DAYS IN
THE FRIDGE

4 tablespoons reduced-fat
 mayonnaise
4 tablespoons nonfat
 buttermilk
½ cup 2% milk
1 ounce Parmigiano-
 Reggiano, grated
¼ teaspoon freshly ground
 black pepper

NUTRITION FACTS

Serving size 2 tablespoons
Servings 8
Calories 52
Calories from Fat 34
Total Fat 4 g (6%)
Saturated Fat 1 g (6%)
Trans Fats 0 g
Monounsaturated Fat 0 g
Cholesterol 7 mg (2%)
Sodium 132 mg (6%)
Total Carbohydrates 2 g (1%)
Dietary Fiber 0 g (0%)
Sugars 2 g
Protein 2 g
Vitamin A (1%)
Vitamin C (0%)
Calcium (7%)
Iron (0%)

*Parenthetical percentages
refer to % Daily Value.

The easiest recipes are always the best. This combines two essential flavors in my kitchen— pepper and Parmigiano—in a rich creamy dressing that takes only a few seconds to make. This dressing is great on salad but is wonderful for sandwiches and wraps!

You do have to use the real thing in this recipe. Cheap imitation Parmesan won't have the rich flavor that makes this dressing.

1. Place all ingredients in a mini chopper or blender and blend until smooth.
2. Chill for at least 1 hour before using.

Myth: Low-fat and fat-free (nonfat) foods are low in calories.

Truth: Eating a lower fat diet is good for you. That said, you must have fat in your diet. Beyond the fact that your body needs fats, they taste good.

It is important to remember that *low-fat* doesn't always mean low calorie, and *nonfat* does not mean no calories. Apples don't have any fat and are good for you, but they still have calories.

The problem is that a lot of low-fat or nonfat foods are actually very high in calories. Many times they are also much higher in sodium than the "regular" version. Food manufacturers will add sugars and other carbohydrates as well as salt to compensate for the fat that is left out.

Always check the calories of foods that you are eating. Many times the low-fat version will have almost the same number of calories (or more) than the full-fat version.

There are some instances where low-fat is generally better. Dairy products are one. On the other hand, any snack food that is labeled low-fat (or low-anything) should be suspect. Check the Nutrition Facts on the label.

Day 38 Alternative Dinner Choices

CONVENIENCE MEALS

Lean Cuisine Spaghetti with Meat Sauce

RESTAURANT MEALS

Noodles and Company House Marinara (small) with Small Side Salad

DAY 39 | LIMIT CONVENIENCE FOODS

You've seen the ads for Nutrisystem. Does it work? Yes (in a way). I do have patients who have lost weight using this plan, and even though it's subjective on my part, it does appear to work well. But not for long.

Why does it work? Planning. First off, the folks at Nutrisystem do the planning for you. You get twenty-one meals per week, supposedly tailored to your life. What you get are meals very much like Lean Cuisine or Weight Watchers frozen meals. What could be wrong with this? Why cook yourself? Convenience meals are so . . . well . . . convenient. Why ever cook again?

Well, the main problem is that most folks get tired of programs like this. Nutrisystem and Jenny Craig are the heavyweights (hee-hee) in the diet plan marketplace, and after time people get tired of the food. Face it, frozen food is only so good for so long. The second problem is that the programs don't really teach you anything. They don't make money helping you learn how to plan for yourself, cook meals, and understand what the right portion sizes are. So when folks stop using these types of plans, they're right back where they started from.

In some ways it's even worse for those who use these plans, because they can't learn portion size from these meals. That's because the portions are small. *Really* small. I've measured these meals and there's not much to them. The 2 ounces of pasta that is a sensible portion for most people is only 1 ounce in most of the plans' diet meals. Likewise, the meat and fish weigh in at only 2 ounces (again, half of what a normal portion should be).

So folks don't learn to plan and they don't learn to cook and they don't come away understanding portion size. So do these frozen convenience meals have a place in your diet at all? Why have I bothered to include them as options in the meal plans here?

Because you're busy. For a lot of us it can be a challenge to cook every night. In the same way that I have given you guidance on what to eat when you go out to restaurants and having items on hand for Pantry Meals, keeping alternatives in your freezer gives you something healthier as part of your plan. Not perfect, mind you, but it's far better than the alternative of ordering from Domino's.

The key is to use convenience meals as *part* of your plan when you know you won't have time for a Pantry Meal or to cook from scratch. When you are using them, make sure that you recognize the difference between the proper portion size of a Dr. Gourmet recipe and the much smaller portion size of the convenience meal.

Find the ones that you like and make sure that you have them stocked in your freezer for those times when you just don't have time. Here's a list of convenience meals that have been reviewed by Dr. Gourmet tasters and come out as being pretty good. You can find complete reviews of each of these and the ones that we didn't like at www.drgourmet.com/reviews/.

Pasta Dishes:

Amy's Garden Vegetable Lasagna

Amy's Rice Mac and Cheese

Amy's Tofu Vegetable Lasagna

Healthy Choice Portabella Marsala Pasta

Healthy Choice Portabella Spinach Parmesan

Healthy Choice Pumpkin Squash Ravioli

Healthy Choice Tomato Basil Penne

Kashi Chicken Florentine

Kashi Chicken Pasta Pomodoro

Lean Cuisine Butternut Squash Ravioli

Lean Cuisine Café Classics Bowl: Grilled Chicken Caesar

Lean Cuisine Chicken in Peanut Sauce

Lean Cuisine Chicken Fettuccini

Lean Cuisine Chicken Parmesan

Lean Cuisine Grilled Chicken with Penne Pasta

Lean Cuisine Macaroni and Cheese

Lean Cuisine Sesame Stir Fry with Chicken

Lean Cuisine Salmon with Basil

Lean Cuisine Spaghetti with Meat Sauce

Lean Cuisine Szechuan Style Stir Fry with Shrimp

Lean Cuisine Three Cheese Stuffed Rigatoni

Michael Angelo's Chicken Parmesan

Michael Angelo's Four Cheese Lasagna

Michael Angelo's Lasagna with Meat Sauce

Michael Angelo's Vegetable Lasagna

Weight Watchers Smart Ones Lasagna Florentine

Weight Watchers Smart Ones Picante Chicken & Pasta

Weight Watchers Spaghetti with Meat Sauce

Weight Watchers Smart Ones Three Cheese Ziti Marinara

Lean Cuisine Macaroni and Cheese

  Mac 'n' Cheese:

365 Macaroni & Cheese

Amy's Country Cheddar Bowl

Amy's Rice Mac and Cheese

Amy's Macaroni & Cheese (frozen)

Annie's Shells & Cheddar

Annie's Whole Wheat Shells and White Cheddar

Lean Cuisine Macaroni and Cheese

Pizza:

Amy's Organic Flour, Broccoli Basil & Tomatoes Pizza Pesto

DiGiorno Harvest Wheat Pizza

DiGiorno Rising Crust Pizza-Three Mushroom

Frontera Frozen Pizzas

Kashi All Natural Mediterranean Pizza

Wolfgang Puck's Grilled Vegetable Cheeseless Pizza

Chili/Soup:

Amy's Organic Chili: Low-Fat Medium Black Bean (gluten free)

Amy's Organic Low Fat Butternut Squash Soup

Amy's Organic Low Fat Cream of Tomato Soup (gluten free)

Campbell's Chunky Healthy Request Chicken Noodle Soup

Campbell's Healthy Request Tomato Soup

Health Valley Chili: Mild Black Bean

Burritos, Pockets, and Sandwiches:

Amy's Black Bean Burrito

Kashi Chicken Rustico Pocket Sandwich

Kashi Turkey Fiesta Pocket Sandwich

Lean Cuisine Chicken, Spinach and Mushroom Panini

Lean Cuisine Southwest Style Chicken Panini

Lean Pockets Ham and Cheddar

Michael Angelo's Pepperoni & Cheese Pocket Calzone

Michael Angelo's Spinach & Vegetable Pocket Calzone

Michael Angelo's Turkey & Cheese Pocket Calzone

Beef:

Healthy Choice Beef Tips Portobello

Michael Angelo's Lasagna with Meat Sauce

Weight Watchers Spaghetti with Meat Sauce (Bolognese)

Chicken/Turkey:

Healthy Choice Grilled Turkey Breast

Healthy Choice Portabella Spinach Parmesan

Kashi Chicken Florentine

Kashi Chicken Pasta Pomodoro

Kashi Chicken Rustico Pocket Sandwich

Kashi Lemongrass Coconut Chicken

Kashi Lemon Rosemary Chicken

Kashi Southwest Style Chicken

Kashi Sweet & Sour Chicken

Kashi Turkey Fiesta Pocket Sandwich

Ethnic Gourmet: Chicken Tandoori

Lean Cuisine Baked Chicken

Lean Cuisine Café Classics Bowl: Grilled Chicken Caesar

Lean Cuisine Chicken in Peanut Sauce

Lean Cuisine Chicken Enchilada Suiza

Lean Cuisine Chicken Parmesan

Lean Cuisine Chicken Fettuccini

Lean Cuisine Fiesta Grilled Chicken with Mexican-Style Rice

Lean Cuisine Ginger Garlic Stir Fry with Chicken

Lean Cuisine Grilled Chicken with Penne Pasta

Lean Cuisine Lemongrass Chicken

Lean Cuisine Orange Chicken

Lean Cuisine Roasted Turkey and Vegetables

Lean Cuisine Sesame Stir Fry with Chicken

Lean Cuisine Sun-Dried Tomato Pesto Chicken

Michael Angelo's Chicken Parmesan

Weight Watchers Smart Ones Chicken Enchilada Suiza

Weight Watchers Smart Ones Picante Chicken & Pasta

Fish/Shrimp:

Lean Cuisine Lemon Pepper Fish

Lean Cuisine Salmon with Basil

Lean Cuisine Szechuan Style Stir Fry with Shrimp

Pork:

South Beach Living Savory Pork

Vegetarian:

Amy's Black Bean and Vegetable Enchiladas

Amy's Brown Rice and Vegetables Bowl

Amy's Brown Rice, Black-Eyed Peas & Veggies Bowl

Amy's Cheese Tamale Verde

Amy's Garden Vegetable Lasagna

Amy's Indian Mattar Paneer

Amy's Indian Palak Paneer

Amy's Indian Vegetable Korma

Amy's Mexican Casserole

Amy's Mexican Tamale Pie

Amy's Rice Mac and Cheese

Amy's Roasted Vegetable Tamale

Amy's Santa Fe Enchilada Bowl

Amy's Shepherd's Pie (and light-in-sodium version)

Amy's Tamale Verde with Black Beans

Amy's Teriyaki Bowl

Amy's Thai Stir-Fry

Amy's Tortilla Casserole

Amy's Shepherd's Pie

Cedarlane Foods Three Layer Enchilada Pie

Ethnic Gourmet: Palak Paneer

Healthy Choice Asian Potstickers

Healthy Choice Portabella Marsala Pasta

Healthy Choice Pumpkin Squash Ravioli

Healthy Choice Tomato Basil Penne

Kashi Black Bean Mango

Lean Cuisine Macaroni and Cheese

Lean Cuisine Linguine Carbonara

Lean Cuisine Penne Pasta with Tomato Basil Sauce

Lean Cuisine Santa Fe Style Rice & Beans

Michael Angelo's Four Cheese Lasagna

Michael Angelo's Vegetable Lasagna

Weight Watchers Smart Ones Santa Fe Style Rice & Beans

Weight Watchers Smart Ones Lasagna Florentine

DAY 39 | DINNER

SWEET RED PEPPER BARBECUE TUNA, CHEESY QUINOA, AND ROASTED CAULIFLOWER

Sweet Red Pepper Barbecue Tuna

SERVINGS: 6 ▮ **SERVING SIZE:** ¼ CUP SAUCE WITH 4 OUNCES TUNA ▮ THIS RECIPE CAN EASILY BE MULTIPLIED ▮ **COOKING TIME:** 30 MINUTES ▮ THE SAUCE KEEPS WELL FOR 72 HOURS IN THE REFRIGERATOR. THE COOKED TUNA MAKES GREAT LEFTOVERS.

2 red bell peppers
2 tablespoons peach preserves
2 tablespoons pure maple syrup
½ cup cider vinegar
1 tablespoon Worcestershire sauce
⅛ teaspoon hot sauce
¼ teaspoon salt
½ teaspoon dry mustard
1 teaspoon chili powder
1 teaspoon paprika
Spray olive or grapeseed oil
6 (4-ounce) tuna steaks

NUTRITION FACTS

Serving size 4 ounces tuna with ¼ cup sauce
Servings 6
Calories 211
Calories from Fat 52
Total Fat 6 g (9%)
Saturated Fat 1 g (7%)
Trans Fats 0 g
Monounsaturated Fat 2 g
Cholesterol 43 mg (14%)
Sodium 179 mg (7%)
Total Carbohydrates 10 g (3%)
Dietary Fiber 1 g (5%)
Sugars 7 g
Protein 27 g
Vitamin A (81%)
Vitamin C (87%)
Calcium (2%)
Iron (10%)

*Parenthetical percentages refer to % Daily Value.

I like this sweet sauce a lot, but it's been toned down a little for this book. If you like spicy food, don't hesitate to add more hot sauce. For the brave, between ½ and 1 teaspoon should be sufficient to make this dish really zing.

You can use bottled roasted red peppers for the barbecue sauce. Make sure that the ones that you purchase are packed in water, and my measurements have shown that one medium-size red bell pepper roasted, peeled, and seeded weighs about 2 ounces. Preparing the sauce the day before makes for a more intense flavor.

If I am cooking more than one serving, I like to cook larger tuna steaks—on the order of 8 to 16 ounces (two to four servings)—then cut them to size before plating. There's less chance of overcooking the tuna that way.

1. Preheat the oven to broil.
2. Place the red pepper in the oven and roast, turning frequently, until blackened on all sides. Remove and place in a brown paper bag. Allow it to cool slightly.
3. Peel and seed the cooled pepper.
4. Place the pepper in a blender with the peach preserves, maple syrup, vinegar, Worcestershire sauce, hot sauce, salt, dry mustard, chili powder, and paprika. Blend until smooth.

5. Preheat oven to 400°F. Place a large ovenproof skillet in the oven. When the oven is hot, spray the pan lightly with oil and add the tuna. (If cooking more than three or four servings, use a second or third skillet. If the tuna is too crowded in the pan, it will not sear properly.)

6. Let the tuna sear for 2 minutes and turn. After 2 minutes, add the barbecue sauce (¼ cup per serving). Cook for another 2 minutes and turn.

7. Cook the tuna for another 2 to 4 minutes and remove from the oven. Slice and serve topped with the remaining sauce.

Chef Tim Says . . . Eat Worcestershire Sauce

Worcestershire sauce has its origins in India. The first attempt by John Lea and William Perrins to re-create the condiment for Western consumers was a failure. That reject was left in the cellar and years later rediscovered. The aging process had transformed their failure into the sauce we now know. (Lea and Perrins' company was in the county of Worcestershire, thus the name of the product.)

The sauce contains vinegar, molasses, cloves, anchovies, tamarind, chili peppers, shallots, garlic, and onion, among other ingredients. It has a great flavor and is very low in sodium.

Cheesy Quinoa

SERVINGS: 2 ▌ SERVING SIZE: ABOUT 1 CUP ▌ THIS RECIPE CAN EASILY BE MULTIPLIED BY UP TO 10 FOR A CROWD ▌ COOKING TIME: 25 MINUTES

½ cup quinoa
½ ounce goat cheese
½ ounce Parmigiano-
    Reggiano, grated
⅛ teaspoon salt

1. Place 2 cups of water in a small saucepan over high heat.

2. When the water boils, add the quinoa. Lower the heat to a high simmer and cover the pan partially. Cook until the water is almost evaporated, stirring occasionally.

3. When the quinoa is just tender, add the goat cheese, Parmesan, and salt. Stir until the cheese is melted and serve.

[CONTINUES]

ITION FACTS

Serving size 1 cup
Servings 2
Calories 203
Calories from Fat 52
Total Fat 6 g (9%)
Saturated Fat 2 g (12%)
Trans Fat 0 g
Monounsaturated Fat 2 g
Cholesterol 8 mg (3%)
Sodium 285 mg (12%)
Total Carbohydrates 28 g (9%)
Dietary Fiber 3 g (12%)
Sugars 0 g
Protein 10 g
Vitamin A (2%)
Vitamin C (0%)
Calcium (11%)
Iron (12%)

*Parenthetical percentages
refer to % Daily Value.

Chef Tim Says . . . Eat Quinoa

Quinoa is a great choice for side dishes and you should keep this grain in your pantry. It has tons of fiber and great texture, with a slightly nutty flavor.

You can use it almost anywhere you would use rice. If you have a favorite rice recipe, quinoa works pretty much the same except your rice recipe is likely 3:1 liquid to rice, whereas 2:1 works with quinoa. Bring the liquid to a boil and add the quinoa. Reduce the heat to a simmer. Unlike rice, you can stir it a bit and it won't get gummy. Stirring will keep your quinoa fluffy.

If you have a rice cooker, the same holds true. Use a 2:1 liquid to quinoa combination (2 cups of water to 1 cup of quinoa). If you don't stir the quinoa, you'll get a little browning at the bottom of the cook pan (depending on how your rice cooker works). I like this and will stir the quinoa just as the rice cooker is done, because it offers a lovely caramelized flavor that enhances the nuttiness of the quinoa.

Roasted Cauliflower

SERVINGS: 2 ▌ **SERVING SIZE:** 4 OUNCES CAULIFLOWER ▌ THIS RECIPE CAN EASILY BE MULTIPLIED ▌ **COOKING TIME:** 25 MINUTES ▌ THIS RECIPE KEEPS WELL IN THE REFRIGERATOR

Spray olive oil
8 ounces cauliflower, broken into small flowerets
1 tablespoon olive oil
⅛ teaspoon dried tarragon
⅛ teaspoon dried marjoram
¼ teaspoon salt
Freshly ground black pepper

I often overlook cauliflower in the market because I am fixed on something "green." Easy and quick and delicious, this is the perfect side dish for almost any meal.

1. Place a large ovenproof skillet in the oven and preheat to 325°F. When the pan is hot, spray lightly with oil and add the cauliflower.

2. Return the pan to the oven and roast the cauliflower for 20 to 25 minutes, tossing occasionally.

3. While the cauliflower is roasting, place the olive oil, tarragon, marjoram, salt, and pepper to taste in a large bowl.

Serving size 4 ounces
   cauliflower
Servings 2
Calories 88
Calories from Fat 61
Total Fat 7 g (11%)
Saturated Fat 1 g (5%)
Trans Fat 0 g
Monounsaturated Fat 5 g
Cholesterol 0 mg (0%)
Sodium 325 mg (14%)
Total Carbohydrates 6 g (2%)
Dietary Fiber 3 g (11%)
Sugars 3 g
Protein 2 g
Vitamin A (0%)
Vitamin C (87%)
Calcium (3%)
Iron (3%)

*Parenthetical percentages
refer to % Daily Value.

4. When the cauliflower is tender, transfer it to the large bowl. Toss to melt the spread and coat the cauliflower, then serve.

Dr. Tim Says . . .

Myth: Skipping a meal is a good way to diet and lose weight.

Truth: Research shows that if you skip meals, you are more likely to be overweight. This appears to be especially true for those who skip breakfast.

When you skip meals, your body slows its metabolism. The theory is that this is to preserve the stored calories through slowing the need for them. There is also good evidence that if you skip a meal, you are likely to eat more at the next one, or worse, to snack (usually on whatever is handy).

Eat three regular meals a day, and if you are working at losing weight, eat smaller portions.

Day 39 Alternative Dinner Choices

CONVENIENCE MEALS

Lean Cuisine Salmon with Basil

RESTAURANT MEALS

P. F. Chang's Oolong Marinated Sea Bass

DAY 40 | EAT HEALTHY WHEN DINING OUT

I spend a lot of time talking with patients about changing their diet and the issue of eating out always comes up. I think going out to eat is an essential part of life and eating healthy. Most of us need to eat out for the sake of convenience. That's why I've included restaurant meals as alternatives in this book.

As with your diet, eating out is about planning. When you are getting ready to go out, choose a place that's going to have healthier options. It's best to avoid fast food, but in an emergency, you can find some okay choices at fast-food restaurants. Although they're supposed to provide the nutritional content of their food in the restaurant, they don't do a very good job. Many, such as chain restaurants Chili's, Applebee's, and Red Lobster, will have their Nutrition Facts online. If they don't provide that information at all, don't eat there. Check before you go, and over time you will build up a list of good choices.

Once again, if you don't know what's in your food, don't eat it. In fact, the meals are often far unhealthier than those at fast-food joints. For instance, many of the dishes at Chili's have over 2,300 mg of sodium in a single serving. That's more than you should have for a whole day!

Your local café or favorite restaurant isn't likely to provide any nutrition information. This is one reason for spending time cooking at home, as well as measuring your food when you do. With that cooking experience, you'll know what a normal portion size looks like.

Patients always tell me that they eat only salad when they are out for dinner. This can be a healthier choice, but it doesn't have to be your only choice. When you do order salad, be sure to ask for the dressing on the side. Dressings can have more than 75 calories in a 2-tablespoon serving.

Looking at almost any restaurant menu, fish is generally a great choice, but be sure that it is grilled, steamed, or poached. The standard restaurant serving of fish is generally about 8 ounces. For lower-calorie diets, this works out to two servings. Keep in mind that 4 ounces of fish or meat is about the size of a deck of cards.

You're not stuck with always eating grilled fish, though. Often your best choice from the menu will be beef. (Surprise!) A lean petit filet mignon may have less fat and calories than chicken. Be careful, though, because chefs love to sauce their dishes: The added calories can be twice what is in the fish or beef. If a sauce is offered, ask for it on the side, and choose a grilled steak such as filet, hanger steak, or sirloin. Many restaurants will list the weight of the steak on the menu, so it'll be easy for you to decide what or how much to eat.

Lastly, don't hesitate to take home a doggie bag. With most restaurants serving twice or more the amount of food you need, you can easily have some for lunch the next day. A patient once shared with me a great idea: Box the half that you aren't going to eat *before* you start to eat your dinner. You won't miss what's not on your plate.

Parties

Going to a party can be a challenge when you're working on eating healthy. It's one thing to splurge when you know exactly what you're eating, but when someone else is doing the cooking, you can consume too many calories in a hurry. On top of that, a lot of us go to parties instead of to dinner and we go on an empty stomach. Just as there are so many ways to consume extra calories, there are a lot of simple ways to avoid packing on the extra calories. Try these strategies:

Eat something healthy before you go. Have an apple or a handful of nuts. Studies have shown that when we "pre-eat" before meals we eat a lot less food. Not going hungry to that holiday party is key to not overeating once there.

Eat on a plate. It's really important to not walk around and nibble endlessly. Get a plate, put your food on it, and eat from the plate. You'll know how much you have taken and are a lot less likely to get more food than you want or need. Get a small plate and fill it no more than twice. A fantastic tip when hosting a party is to make sure that you provide smaller plates for your guests so they'll have a choice.

So . . . what to put on that plate? If there are roasted meats, they'll be a great choice. These are usually lean and really tasty. Shrimp cocktail is a good choice for the same reason. Take all the veggies that you want— they're fantastic for you and will help fill you up on great tasting food. There's always some dip to go with them. Put a couple of spoonfuls on your plate and dip from there. Nuts are always a fine choice as a snack and this is especially true at the cocktail party. They are filling, good for you, and taste great.

Don't put anything on your plate that's been fried. Steer clear of savory pastries—just one of those pigs in a blanket can be up to 150 calories for a single bite or two, and it's not filling. Those little mini-quiches and other pastries are just as chock full of fat and calories. You can eat a plate full of shrimp and not get as many calories.

Stick to real food. I always talk about nuts because I know that they're so good for you, whereas all those crackers, chips, and pretzels are empty calories. Avoid the junk food. One note of caution, however: Don't eat the sugared nuts that are so popular at the holidays.

If there are more substantial hors d'oeuvres, party foods can be an okay substitute for dinner, but choose carefully. There will often be chafing dishes filled with foods that are heavily sauced. Simply put the lid back and move on.

Eat one or two bite-size desserts, then stop. The nice thing about many parties is that the desserts have often been laid out in bite sizes. If there are desserts, take a small piece and enjoy it. This is another good place to use a plate. Make a trip to the dessert table, put one or two on your plate, and enjoy! (Then stop.)

Don't drink on an empty stomach. For a lot of folks, alcohol is part of the party—especially at the holidays. Drink if you like, but don't drink on an empty stomach. Have a plate of veggies with some dip first and then get a glass of wine. Set your limit of drinks at a healthy two or at the most three. A good way is to alternate cocktails or wine with sparkling or mineral water. Keep track of how much you drink.

Skip the egg nog. If you like egg nog, do be careful. Most egg nog recipes have tons and tons of calories. A cup can have as much as 400 calories so it's best to have a few sips and go back to your wine.

DAY 40 | DINNER

LEFTOVER SPAGHETTI AND MEATBALLS (PAGE 232) AND SALAD WITH PARMESAN PEPPERCORN DRESSING (PAGE 234)

Day 40 Alternative Dinner Choices

CONVENIENCE MEALS

Lean Cuisine Spaghetti with Meat Sauce

RESTAURANT MEALS

Noodles and Company House Marinara (small) with Small Side Salad

DAY 41 | EAT HEALTHY WHEN YOU TRAVEL

I will often have patients remark on how they can't eat healthy while they're traveling. This comes both from people who only travel occasionally, for pleasure, as well as those who make a living on the road. Just like at home, planning is the essential. Thinking about what and when you are going to eat beforehand makes all the difference.

I spend a fair amount of time traveling, both for Dr. Gourmet as well as for pleasure. The one good thing about business travel is that it is predictable—we know where we are going to be and are able to research that. As with other travel, attending a wedding or other special occasion is an opportunity for overindulgence, but you can eat well and eat healthy with a bit of planning.

Before you go, do a Google search of the area where you're staying. Put in the hotel address and the words "healthy food" and you'll find plenty of choices. Another alternative is the booking service OpenTable.com. Or look on ChowHound.com or Chow.com. There are often great suggestions on the forums.

Snacks

Packing snacks in your bag can save you when you can't find any healthy meals. Road warriors are often up early for meetings before even the hotel restaurant is open. Having nuts, trail mix, or even a granola bar provides you with a great alternative and you won't be hungry when you pass by the doughnuts as they speak to you: "You're hungry, aren't you? Eat us! Go on, just one."

I always travel with things like fruit, nuts, granola bars, trail mix, and bottles of water. When the snack on the plane is offered, or if I can't find something good for breakfast or lunch, I always have something better for me that also tastes a lot better.

Breakfast

Focus on breakfast; it's key to not being hungry later. If you're leaving on an early flight, get up and have something, even if it's quick. A bowl of whole-grain cereal or oatmeal that's high in fiber will stay with you and keep you from being hungry later.

Even if you're in a hurry, make up a bagel with a little light cream cheese or jam and take it with you to eat on the plane. Toss in a banana or an apple (or even pick up some fruit in the terminal). And you don't have to have "breakfast." A peanut butter sandwich is the perfect on the go meal.

The same holds true for when you are on the road. Make sure to get up early to have breakfast. Check the menu at your hotel. A lot of hotels offer free continental breakfast with healthy cereal and fruit choices. One of the best bowls of steel-cut oatmeal I have ever had was in a hotel dining room in the middle of Yosemite.

Lunch

Lunch while traveling can be a challenge because most of us jump into the closest fast-food joint. Eating breakfast will help you avoid being hungry, but the trick is to be prepared to have something healthier.

Salad is an obvious choice for a healthy lunch, and looking for a salad bar makes sense (but be careful with the dressing).

Starbucks has some good prepared meals, including a cheese and fruit plate and pasta salads.

Look for wraps as a portable alternative. These are easily carried and a veggie wrap can be a great choice that you can pick up on the way to the plane. Use the restaurant guide on the Dr. Gourmet Web site.

Sandwiches can be a decent choice and Subway is pretty good because the nutrition information on their sandwiches is listed in every restaurant. They also have whole wheat bread. But be careful, because some sandwiches are really high in calories.

Dinner

When I travel, I like to try to find a Mediterranean restaurant. The great thing about Greek, Lebanese, or Turkish food is that there are usually meze choices. These are small plates, such as stuffed grape leaves, hummus, or baba ganoush. It's easy to overeat in any restaurant, so consider ordering two or three appetizers instead of a full main course. You'll not only eat less but be able to sample more great food. Alternatively, I look for fish choices, grilled or broiled with simple sauces, on the restaurant menu.

Eat breakfast, plan for lunch, carry snacks, and choose meze plates or grilled fish for dinner. Think about where you are going and what you are going to eat ahead of time. You *can* eat great food and eat healthy on the road.

Chef Tim Says . . . Eat Capers

Capers are the flower bud of a bush from the family *Capparidaceae*. Cultivated in the hot climates of the Mediterranean and Asia, the immature flowers are picked and then pickled in vinegar brine. They are bland when raw, but pickled capers are pungent with a sharp piquant flavor. They are high in antioxidants and almost calorie free (1 tablespoon = 2 calories). Capers can add a lot of salt (and salty flavor) to dishes, with a teaspoon having about 80 mg sodium, but they are so flavorful a little goes a long way.

DAY 41 | DINNER

SALMON WITH CAPER MAYONNAISE AND SAVORY QUINOA

Salmon with Caper Mayonnaise

SERVINGS: 4 ▌ **SERVING SIZE:** 4 OUNCES SALMON AND 1½ TABLESPOONS MAYONNAISE ▌ THIS RECIPE IS EASILY MULTIPLIED ▌ **COOKING TIME:** 30 MINUTES ▌ THE MAYONNAISE KEEPS WELL FOR ABOUT 3 DAYS. THE LEFTOVER FISH MAKES GREAT SANDWICHES.

¼ cup reduced-fat
    mayonnaise
2 tablespoons fresh curly
    parsley, minced
½ teaspoon dried tarragon
1 tablespoon freshly
    squeezed lemon juice
2 tablespoons capers
4 (4-ounce) salmon fillets

NUTRITION FACTS

Serving size 4 ounces salmon
    with 1½ tablespoons
    mayonnaise
Servings 4
Calories 243
Calories from Fat 132
Total Fat 15 g (23%)
Saturated Fat 2 g (12%)
Trans Fat 0 g
Monounsaturated Fat 5 g
Cholesterol 75 mg (25%)
Sodium 300 mg (12%)
Total Carbohydrates 2 g (1%)
Dietary Fiber <1 g (1%)
Sugars 1 g
Protein 24 g
Vitamin A (8%)
Vitamin C (6%)
Calcium (1%)
Iron (4%)

*Parenthetical percentages
refer to % Daily Value.

I like grilled salmon so much, and to put anything on it is a bit like gilding the lily, but this mayonnaise is so versatile. You can use most any herb that you like—chives, thyme, basil.

1. Mix the mayonnaise, parsley, tarragon, lemon juice, and capers and chill.

2. Preheat the oven to broil. Place the salmon fillets on a nonstick cookie sheet.

3. Place under the broiler and cook for about 5 minutes.

4. Top with 2 tablespoons of the herbed mayonnaise and return to the broiler for another 5 minutes, until the salmon is just cooked through.

Dr. Tim Says . . . Eat Reduced-Fat Mayonnaise

The amount of fat varies pretty widely between nonfat and regular mayonnaise, the latter of which has up to 10 to 11 grams of fat per tablespoon.

Reduced-fat mayonnaises are great for making salads, and there are a number of choices available to you. I feel that Best Foods and Hellman's reduced-fat mayonnaise has far and away the best flavor, with only 2 grams of fat and 25 calories per tablespoon.

I don't like using nonfat mayonnaise for dressings—I have found that they simply aren't creamy enough. For a recipe like Red Pepper Mayonnaise, however, fat-free is perfect because the other ingredients make for a rich flavor.

Light mayonnaise or reduced-fat mayonnaise usually has about 2 grams of fat per tablespoon. I generally keep this around for making sandwiches.

Savory Quinoa

SERVINGS: 2 ▌ **SERVING SIZE:** ABOUT 1 CUP ▌ THIS RECIPE CAN EASILY BE MULTIPLIED
▌ **COOKING TIME:** 30 MINUTES ▌ THIS RECIPE DOES NOT MAKE VERY GOOD LEFTOVERS

1 teaspoon olive oil
1 large shallot, minced
2 cloves garlic, minced
1 rib celery, diced
½ cup quinoa
¼ teaspoon salt
Freshly ground black
     pepper
1 cup no-salt-added chicken
     stock

NUTRITION FACTS

Serving size 1 cup
Servings 2
Calories 223
Calories from Fat 50
Total Fat 6 g (9%)
Saturated Fat 1 g (4%)
Trans Fat 0 g
Monounsaturated Fat 2 g
Cholesterol 0 mg (0%)
Sodium 349 mg (15%)
Total Carbohydrates 35 g (12%)
Dietary Fiber 3 g (13%)
Sugars 1 g
Protein 9 g
Vitamin A (9%)
Vitamin C (6%)
Calcium (5%)
Iron (15%)

*Parenthetical percentages
refer to % Daily Value.

The nuttiness of the quinoa and the savory shallots and chicken stock complement each other just right.

1. Place the olive oil in a medium-size saucepan over medium-high heat. Add the shallot and garlic. Cook, stirring frequently, for about 3 minutes.

2. Add the celery and cook for another 2 minutes.

3. Add the quinoa, salt, and pepper. Cook, stirring continuously, for about 1 minute.

4. Add the chicken stock and 1 cup of water. When the water boils, lower the heat until the quinoa is simmering. Stir occasionally.

5. Cook until the quinoa is soft and the liquid evaporated. Add more water ¼ cup at a time, if needed. The total cooking time is 25 to 30 minutes.

CONVENIENCE MEALS

Lean Cuisine Salmon with Basil

RESTAURANT MEALS

Red Lobster Grilled Fish with Baked Potato and a Side Salad

DAY 42 | *GET YOUR VITAMINS FROM REAL FOODS, NOT SUPPLEMENTS*

There are so many vitamins and supplements on the market now, and they just seem so promising: Take a pill and be healthier. Unfortunately, for the most part, they simply don't work. It's becoming clear from research that all those pills, capsules, and supplement drinks are worthless and you don't need a multivitamin to be healthy. The research does show that you need vitamins and will be healthier for getting them in your diet, but only when you get them from your food. Think quality calories!

One study evaluated the effect of vitamin C on inflammation.[10] The study set out to answer whether eating foods high in vitamin C would have an effect on inflammatory markers in the blood. It was clear that a higher intake of vitamin C from fruits resulted in a lower amount of inflammation. Vitamin C intake from veggies showed reduced blood-clotting factors. Unfortunately, the research using vitamin supplements does not show the same results.

Research from the National Institutes of Health, looking at vitamin C consumption in healthy adults, shows that the current RDA of 60 mg of vitamin C daily may not be enough.[11] Recommended Daily Allowances (RDAs) were originally designed to prevent vitamin deficiencies, and scientists are rethinking that strategy. The new recommendation is that 100 to 200 mg of vitamin C each day will best meet most adult needs. The same research showed that consuming more than 1,000 mg daily was found to be detrimental (people often do this using supplements). It's easy to meet these new RDAs by eating five servings of fruits or vegetables per day. (Keep in mind that you really *can't* eat too many fruits and veggies.) Most people think only citrus fruits such as oranges and grapefruit are high in vitamin C, but you'll get a lot in almost any fruit you choose.

Studies on supplements just haven't shown promising benefits. In one well-designed study, researchers used a supplement containing eleven vitamins and five minerals. Participants were given either the test supplement or a placebo to take every day for a year.[12] Their mental status was assessed at the beginning and the end of the study, using standard tests. Results showed no difference between the two groups' mental abilities at the end of the study.

In a large analysis of eleven different studies, researchers looked at whether taking supplements of antioxidants and B vitamins would affect the progression of heart disease.[13] The research evaluated the amount of plaque lining the arteries of the heart. There was no evidence that taking vitamins in pill form had any effect on the buildup of plaque, and six of the studies suggested that antioxidants in pill form might actually make the heart disease worse. Even worse, the supplements appeared to reduce the effects of beneficial heart medications.

An excellent comprehensive study recently looked at vitamin E and selenium, specifically at whether taking both could prevent prostate cancer.[14] The study evaluated a variety of combinations of these two supplements, and found that alone or in combination, neither had any effect on the prevention of prostate cancer.

Another very large study released in 2008 by a group that specializes in such research demonstrated that the available information indicates no benefit from antioxidant preparations.[15] They showed, in fact, that those products might actually harm you.

It's clear that the best way to get your vitamins is by eating healthy foods.

There is one exception to the research. It is felt that women of childbearing age should take a daily multivitamin. This is because multivitamins are required to contain 400 micrograms of folic acid. Also known as folate, this is essential to normal formation of the embryo in the first few weeks after conception, and a diet low in folic acid can result in a fetus with spina bifida, an extremely serious defect of the spine or brain.

Good Sources of Vitamin A:
Turkey
Carrots
Sweet potatoes
Spinach
Collard greens
Kale
Turnip greens
Winter squash
Red peppers
Cantaloupe

Good Sources of Vitamin D:
Catfish
Oysters
Salmon
Trout
Halibut
Sardines
Mackerel
Shrimp
Tuna fish
Milk fortified with vitamin D
Orange juice fortified with vitamin D

Good Sources of Vitamin C:
Orange juice
Red peppers
Green peppers
Grapefruit
Peaches
Papayas
Broccoli
Peas
Sweet potatoes
Strawberries

Good Sources of Vitamin E:
Sunflower seeds
Almonds
Spinach
Tomatoes
Soy milk
Pumpkin
Crab
Broccoli
Red peppers
Rockfish

Pizza with Tomato, Basil, and Roasted Garlic

SERVINGS: 1 ▌ SERVING SIZE: 1 INDIVIDUAL PIZZA ▌ THIS RECIPE CAN EASILY BE MULTI-
PLIED BY 2, 3, OR 4 ▌ LEFTOVERS ARE GOOD COLD FOR BREAKFAST ▌ COOKING TIME:
90 MINUTES

1 medium-size (4 ounce) tomato, seeded and sliced vertically into ¼-inch strips
1 ounce fresh mozzarella, cut into ½-inch cubes
8 large fresh basil leaves, cut into chiffonade
4 cloves Roasted Garlic (recipe follows), quartered
½ ounce Parmigiano-Reggiano, grated
¼ recipe Whole Wheat Pizza Dough (page 55)

NUTRITION FACTS

Serving size 1 pizza (includes dough & toppings)
Servings 1
Calories 479
Calories from Fat 109
Total Fat 12 g (19%)
Saturated Fat 6 g (32%)
Trans Fats 0 g
Monounsaturated Fat 4 g
Cholesterol 32 mg (11%)
Sodium 708 mg (30%)
Total Carbohydrates 73 g (24%)
Dietary Fiber 10 g (40%)
Sugars 11 g
Protein 24 g
Vitamin A (13%)
Vitamin C (35%)
Calcium (41%)
Iron (31%)

*Parenthetical percentages refer to % Daily Value.

This is one of my favorite pizzas. The combination of the roasted garlic, fresh mozzarella, tomatoes, and basil is perfect together. It may seem strange to have pizza without sauce, but the fresh ingredients make this rich and flavorful. This recipe requires that the Whole Wheat Pizza Dough (see page 55) and Roasted Garlic (recipe follows) be made first.

1. Preheat the oven to 500°F. Pizza is best baked on a pizza stone, but a cookie sheet will work as well. Place the baking stone or cookie sheet in the oven and allow it to heat at least 15 to 20 minutes.

2. Gently toss the tomato strips, mozzarella, basil leaves, and garlic together in a small mixing bowl.

3. Set the tomato mixture close to the oven so that it will be accessible and easy to place on top of the dough. Have the grated Parmesan within easy reach.

4. Using one-quarter of the pizza dough recipe (for each pizza), gently stretch into 8-inch rounds. Don't work too hard to get a perfectly round shape.

5. Once the dough is formed, place on the hot pizza stone and top with the tomato mixture.

6. Bake for about 8 minutes, then top with the Parmesan. Bake for another 3 to 5 minutes, until the cheese has melted. Remove from the oven and let cool for about 90 seconds, then slice and serve.

Roasted Garlic

SERVINGS: 6 ▮ **SERVING SIZE:** ⅓ HEAD OF GARLIC (ABOUT 6 CLOVES) ▮ I MAKE UP TO FOUR HEADS OF GARLIC AT A TIME ▮ **COOKING TIME:** 30 MINUTES ▮ THIS KEEPS WELL, TIGHTLY COVERED, FOR 4 TO 6 DAYS

2 heads whole garlic
2 teaspoons extra-virgin
  olive oil

NUTRITION FACTS

Serving size ⅓ head of garlic
  (about 4 cloves)
Servings 6
Calories 40
Calories from Fat 14
Total Fat 2 g (2%)
Saturated Fat 0 g (1%)
Trans Fat 0 g
Monounsaturated Fat 0 g
Cholesterol 0 mg (0%)
Sodium 3 mg (0%)
Total Carbohydrates 6 g (2%)
Dietary Fiber 0 g (2%)
Sugars 0 g
Protein 1 g
Vitamin A (0%)
Vitamin C (9%)
Calcium (3%)
Iron (2%)

*Parenthetical percentages
refer to % Daily Value.

Roasted garlic is a staple in my kitchen and should be in yours. I generally roast about three heads every ten days or so. It makes a great ingredient in mashed potatoes and also enriches any sauce. It is fantastic served as hors d'oeuvres on bread with some soft goat cheese and veggies.

1. Preheat the oven to 300°F.

2. Peel the outermost skin of the garlic only. Turn each bulb on its side and slice ½ inch of the stem end, leaving the rest of the bulb whole.

3. Pour the olive oil in the bottom of a heavy-bottomed sauce pan. Place the garlic cut side down in the pan.

4. Cover and roast for 45 minutes, until the cloves are slightly brown at the cut end and soft throughout.

Day 42 Alternative Dinner Choices

DiGiorno Rising Crust Three Mushroom Pizza

Pizza Hut Half-Serving Cheese Only Personal Pan Pizza

Chef Tim Says . . . Eat Fresh Mozzarella

Mozzarella is one of the cheeses the Italians call *pasta filata*—cheeses that have been scalded and kneaded prior to ageing. Ricotta and provolone are also *pasta filata* cheeses. Originally made in Naples from the rich milk of water buffalos, cheeses available outside of Italy that are labeled *mozzarella* can be made from any type of milk.

The most familiar mozzarella to Americans is the low-moisture version. This was created to cater not just to the American palate, but also to satisfy the transportation and storage issues of manufacturers. It is a moist cheese when compared to others traditionally eaten in the United States, but it has a rubbery quality. Even so, it does melt exceptionally well, making it ideally suited for pizza.

A wide variety of high-moisture mozzarellas are available. Much is imported, but many artisan cheese makers are producing amazing products. Most mozzarellas, produced both inside and outside of Italy, are made with cow's milk, usually skim or low fat.

High-moisture mozzarella is often called "fresh" mozzarella. It is soft, with a sublime taste. Look for a cheese that has a soft creamy texture and a taste that evokes fresh milk.

CHAPTER 7 | WEEKS 7 AND 8

MORE GREAT MEAL IDEAS (AND DESSERT)

Quick Tacos (Pantry Meal)

SERVINGS: 2 ▌ **SERVING SIZE:** 3 TACOS ▌ THIS RECIPE CAN EASILY BE MULTIPLIED ▌
COOKING TIME: 30 MINUTES

1 (15-ounce) can no-salt-added diced tomatoes
½ teaspoon ground cumin
¼ teaspoon paprika
½ teaspoon dried oregano
¼ teaspoon chili powder
⅛ teaspoon red pepper flakes (optional)
¼ teaspoon salt
Freshly ground black pepper
1 cup no-salt-added frozen corn kernels
3 ounces reduced-fat cheddar or Monterey Jack cheese, grated
6 trans fat–free taco shells

NUTRITION FACTS

Serving size 3 tacos
Servings 2
Calories 309
Calories from Fat 93
Total Fat 10 g (16%)
Saturated Fat 3 g (17%)
Trans Fat 0 g
Monounsaturated Fat 5 g
Cholesterol 9 mg (3%)
Sodium 687 mg (29%)
Total Carbohydrates 41 g (14%)
Dietary Fiber 5 g (19%)
Sugars 5 g
Protein 16 g
Vitamin A (12%)
Vitamin C (20%)
Calcium (25%)
Iron (15%)

*Parenthetical percentages refer to % Daily Value.

The idea of Pantry Meals is to keep items in your pantry or fridge on hand that can be quickly put together for a great meal. With tacos, if you have an onion, it's easy to dice it and add it to the tomatoes instead of the corn, for instance. Have some fresh lettuce or cilantro on hand? That'll go well also. The key is to have the fundamentals in the house that you can use to make a quick, healthy meal.

Do keep in mind that many of the most popular taco shells on the market, including Old El Paso, contain trans fats. Check the package and purchase only those that don't have any trans fats, such as Taco Bell (made by Kraft) and Casa Fiesta.

The filling for the tacos will keep well for a few days in the refrigerator.

1. Place the diced tomatoes in a medium-size skillet over medium heat.

2. Add the cumin, paprika, oregano, chili powder, red pepper flakes, salt, and pepper to taste. Cook, stirring occasionally, for about 15 minutes.

3. As the tomatoes cook, the liquid will reduce and the tomatoes will thicken. At that point, add the corn and cook for 3 to 5 minutes.

4. Divide the grated cheese into two small piles. Using one pile, place a small amount of cheese in the bottom of each taco shell, dividing the cheese evenly among the six tacos.

5. Add equal amounts of the tomato mixture to the six tacos.

6. Top the taco filling with the remaining cheese, divided evenly among the six tacos. Serve.

Kung Pao Chicken

SERVINGS: 4 ▌ **SERVING SIZE:** 4 OUNCES CHICKEN WITH VEGETABLES AND RICE ▌
THIS RECIPE CAN EASILY BE MULTIPLIED ▌ **COOKING TIME:** 30 MINUTES

2 tablespoons plus 2
    teaspoons low-sodium
    soy sauce
2 teaspoons sake or sweet
    white wine
1 tablespoon plus
    1 teaspoon sesame oil
2 teaspoons rice vinegar
2 teaspoons honey
1 teaspoon cornstarch
16 ounces boneless, skinless
    chicken breast, cut into
    1-inch cubes
1 cup uncooked jasmine rice
2 cloves garlic, minced
1 (1-inch) piece fresh ginger,
    peeled and minced
1 small red chile pepper,
    seeded and minced
4 green onions, cut finely
    crosswise and
    separated into white
    and green parts
2 tablespoons rice vinegar
¼ cup dry-roasted peanuts,
    chopped coarsely

I like spicy food, but not too spicy. This is literally the one-pepper version and is pretty mild. It's easy to make this spicier by adding peppers to your desired level of heat.

One way to control the spice level in dishes like this one is to use chili oil. It adds the flavor of a spicy chile pepper, but you don't have to take the time to seed and mince. Chili oil is widely available now—your grocery store probably carries it—and very common in Asian markets. Simply replace with the chili oil some of the oil that you use to stir-fry. Start slowly at first—½ teaspoon for two servings may be enough for you (it is for me). Each time you cook, use a little more if you want more heat.

This recipe makes great leftovers.

1. Place the 2 teaspoons of soy sauce, sake, 1 teaspoon of sesame oil, vinegar, honey, and the cornstarch in a bowl and stir until well blended. Add the chicken cubes and toss until coated. Place the bowl in the refrigerator.

2. While the chicken is marinating, place 2 cups of water in a medium-size saucepan over high heat. When the water boils, stir in the jasmine rice.

3. Lower the heat to medium-low and simmer, partially covered, for about 15 minutes. Do not boil away all of the liquid and do not stir the rice. When a very small amount of liquid remains, remove the pan from the burner and let it stand, covered, for 5 minutes before serving.

[CONTINUES]

NUTRITION FACTS

Serving size 4 ounces chicken
    with vegetables and rice
Servings 4
Calories 416
Calories from Fat 102
Total Fat 12 g (18%)
Saturated Fat 2 g (10%)
Trans Fat 0 g
Monounsaturated Fat 4 g
Cholesterol 65 mg (22%)
Sodium 367 mg (16%)
Total Carbohydrates 44 g (15%)
Dietary Fiber 3 g (12%)
Sugars 4 g
Protein 33 g
Vitamin A (4%)
Vitamin C (10%)
Calcium (5%)
Iron (13%)

*Parenthetical percentages
refer to % Daily Value.

4. When the rice is done, place a large skillet or wok over high heat. Add the remaining tablespoon of sesame oil and heat for a few moments. Lower the heat to medium and add the garlic, ginger, and chile pepper, and the white part of the green onions. Cook for about 1 minute.

5. Add the chicken and cook for about 1 minute, until browned on the outside.

6. Add the rice vinegar and the remaining 2 tablespoons of soy sauce. Cook the chicken, tossing frequently. When the chicken is nearly done, fold in the green part of the green onion.

7. Serve over the rice and top with the peanuts.

Shrimp Étouffée

SERVINGS: 4 ▌ **SERVING SIZE:** 4 OUNCES SHRIMP ▌ THIS RECIPE CAN BE HALVED OR MULTIPLIED ▌ **COOKING TIME:** 60 MINUTES

6 tablespoons all-purpose flour
2 teaspoons unsalted butter
2 teaspoons olive oil
4 cloves garlic, minced
2 cups diced yellow onions
1 cup diced celery
½ cup seeded and diced green bell peppers
½ cup seeded and diced red bell peppers
½ teaspoon salt
¼ teaspoon freshly ground black pepper
Pinch of cayenne
2 bay leaves
2 teaspoons Cajun spice
1 cup peeled, seeded, and chopped tomatoes
2 tablespoons dry sherry or dry white wine
2 tablespoons fresh parsley, chopped
2 teaspoons fresh thyme, chopped
1 pound shrimp, peeled and deveined
3 tablespoons chopped green onions

A roux is traditionally made with equal parts of flour and a fat. It takes about a tablespoon of flour to thicken a cup of liquid for sauce. But the tablespoon of fat that goes along with the flour adds over a hundred calories to a single cup of sauce. With a brown roux, the flour is allowed to cook longer in the fat, slowly browning the flour. This adds a nutty flavor that is essential in many recipes—especially Cajun and Creole food.

Leftovers are good for 24 to 48 hours. Reheat gently.

1. Place the flour in a large nonstick skillet and heat over medium-high heat. Watching the pan carefully, stir and shake the flour. It will take 10 to 15 minutes for the flour to turn an almond brown. Do not let it cook too fast or burn. Transfer to a plate and let cool.

2. While the flour is cooling, place the butter and olive oil in the pan over medium heat and add the minced garlic. Cook, stirring frequently, until the garlic softens. Add the onion, celery, and green and red peppers and cook until the peppers are slightly soft.

3. Sprinkle about one-quarter of the cooked flour over the top of the cooked vegetables. Stir to blend and repeat, adding the flour in three more batches, until it is fully incorporated and there are no clumps of flour.

[CONTINUES]

NUTRITION FACTS

Serving size about 2 cups/
    4 ounces shrimp (rice not
    included)
Servings 4
Calories 280
Calories from Fat 59
Total Fat 7 g (10%)
Saturated Fat 2 g (10%)
Trans Fats 0 g
Monounsaturated Fat 3 g
Cholesterol 178 mg (59%)
Sodium 784 mg (33%)
Total Carbohydrates 27 g (9%)
Dietary Fiber 4 g (15%)
Sugars 8 g
Protein 27 g
Vitamin A (33%)
Vitamin C (121%)
Calcium (13%)
Iron (26%)

*Parenthetical percentages
refer to % Daily Value.

4. Add 2 cups of water slowly, stirring continuously. The sauce will begin to thicken. Stir in the salt, pepper, cayenne, bay leaves, and Cajun spice.

5. Cook slowly, adding water a tablespoon at a time if the sauce is too thick. Add the tomatoes, sherry, parsley, and thyme. The sauce can be made to this point and kept warm or refrigerated overnight. When ready to serve, heat the sauce and add the shrimp. Cook until they are pink and firm.

6. Serve over brown rice and top with the chopped green onions.

Cajun Cheeseburger

SERVINGS: 2 ▌ **SERVING SIZE:** 1 BURGER ▌ THIS RECIPE CAN EASILY BE MULTIPLIED ▌
COOKING TIME: 30 MINUTES

8 ounces 95% lean ground beef
¼ teaspoon salt
Freshly ground black pepper
2 teaspoons salt-free Cajun/Creole spice blend
¼ cup seeded and finely diced green bell pepper
¼ cup finely diced onion
Spray oil
1½ ounces part–skim milk mozzarella cheese, sliced thinly
2 whole wheat hamburger buns
2 tablespoons reduced-fat mayonnaise

NUTRITION FACTS

Serving size 4-ounce burger
Servings 2
Calories 367
Calories from Fat 113
Total Fat 13 g (19%)
Saturated Fat 6 g (28%)
Trans Fat 0 g
Monounsaturated Fat 4 g
Cholesterol 82 mg (27%)
Sodium 526 mg (22%)
Total Carbohydrates 30 g (10%)
Dietary Fiber 5 g (20%)
Sugars 7 g
Protein 34 g
Vitamin A (11%)
Vitamin C (29%)
Calcium (23%)
Iron (25%)

*Parenthetical percentages refer to % Daily Value.

The first time I made these burgers, they were on the salty side. While I am more sensitive to sodium content than some people are, it seemed odd because I hadn't added that much salt. That's when my wife checked the can of Creole spice I was using. Tony Chachere's is a popular brand in New Orleans and I had used their salt-free seasoning before, but in stews and such.

A look at the can showed that it used potassium as a salt substitute. A check of my other brands in the house, including Paul Prudhomme, McCormick, and Spice Hunter, showed that they were salt and potassium free—just spices.

The third time, using the no-salt/no-potassium version, was the charm with a great burger that's not too salty. It just goes to show, however, just how important reading food labels can be.

1. Preheat the oven to 375°F. Place a medium-size ovenproof skillet in the oven.

2. Place the ground beef in a small mixing bowl and add the salt, pepper, and 1 teaspoon of the Creole/Cajun spice mix. Using a fork, blend in the seasonings well. Add the remaining teaspoon of spice with the bell pepper and onion. Blend well.

3. Divide the ground beef in half and pat into two patties.

4. When the oven is hot, spray the pan lightly with oil.

[CONTINUES]

5. Add the burgers to the pan. Cook for about 5 minutes on one side and turn. Top each with half of the sliced cheese and cook for about another 5 minutes.

6. Serve on the hamburger bun with mayonnaise. Top with lettuce, tomato, and onion as desired.

DAY 46 | DINNER

French Fries

SERVINGS: 4 ▌ SERVING SIZE: ABOUT 4 OUNCES FRIES ▌ THIS RECIPE CAN EASILY BE DOUBLED, BUT MUST BE COOKED IN TWO BATCHES ▌ COOKING TIME: 25 MINUTES

1 pound russet potatoes, peeled and cut into ¼-inch strips
1 quart chilled water
1 tray ice cubes
½ teaspoon salt
Spray canola oil

NUTRITION FACTS

Serving size about 4 ounces
Servings 4
Calories 86
Calories from Fat 1
Total Fat 0 g (0%)
Saturated Fat 0 g (0%)
Trans Fats 0 g
Monounsaturated Fat 0 g
Cholesterol 0 mg (0%)
Sodium 297 mg (12%)
Total Carbohydrates 20 g (7%)
Dietary Fiber 2 g (10%)
Sugars 1 g
Protein 2 g
Vitamin A (0%)
Vitamin C (37%)
Calcium (1%)
Iron (5%)

*Parenthetical percentages refer to % Daily Value.

Oven-fried foods taste just like deep-fried ones, if you handle them right. Most of the time, however, you have to eat the dish right away. These French fries, for instance, will keep for all of about 20 minutes (about the same amount of time as ones that have been deep-fried).

1. After the potatoes are peeled and sliced, place them in a mixing bowl with the cold water and ice cubes. Soak for 30 minutes.

2. Preheat the oven to 400°F.

3. After soaking the potatoes, drain them and then pat dry with a paper towel.

4. Place the potatoes and salt in a zippered plastic bag. Spray the potatoes for about 3 seconds with the canola oil and seal the zipper. Shake to coat the potatoes well with the oil and salt.

5. Carefully place the potatoes on a nonstick cookie sheet. Don't allow the fries to touch one another. Spray lightly with the canola oil.

6. Place the cookie sheet in the oven and allow the potatoes to bake for about 7 minutes. Turn the potatoes at least twice, cooking for about 7 minutes after each turn. The total cooking time will be 20 to 25 minutes.

7. Serve immediately.

LEFTOVER SHRIMP ÉTOUFFÉE (PAGE 265)

Crab Cakes

SERVINGS: 4 ▌ SERVING SIZE: 2 CRAB CAKES ▌ THIS RECIPE CAN EASILY BE MULTIPLIED ▌ COOKING TIME: 30 MINUTES ▌ THE CRAB MIXTURE MAY BE PREPARED UP TO 12 HOURS IN ADVANCE

1 pound lump crabmeat, picked over to remove any shells
⅓ cup low-sodium saltine crackers, broken into ¼-inch pieces
½ teaspoon Tabasco sauce
2 teaspoons Worcestershire sauce
1 tablespoon shallot, minced
2 teaspoons Dijon mustard
1 large egg white
1 rib celery, diced
1 tablespoon fresh lemon juice
2 tablespoons reduced-fat mayonnaise
⅛ teaspoon salt
Freshly ground black pepper
2 teaspoons extra-virgin olive oil

NUTRITION FACTS

Serving size 2 crab cakes
Servings 4
Calories 168
Calories from Fat 55
Total Fat 6 g (9%)
Saturated Fat 1 g (5%)
Trans Fats 0 g
Monounsaturated Fat 2 g
Cholesterol 90 mg (30%)
Sodium 491 mg (20%)
Total Carbohydrates 5 g (2%)
Dietary Fiber <1 g (1%)
Sugars 1 g
Protein 22 g
Vitamin A (1%)
Vitamin C (9%)
Calcium (11%)
Iron (8%)

*Parenthetical percentages refer to % Daily Value.

Cooked crab cakes will make good sandwiches the next day.

1. Fold the crabmeat together with the crumbled saltines. Add the Tabasco sauce, Worcestershire sauce, shallot, mustard, egg white, celery, lemon juice, mayonnaise, salt, and pepper. Fold together gently until well blended. Be careful to not break up the crabmeat too much.

2. Form into eight cakes and chill for up to 12 hours.

3. Preheat the oven to 400°F.

4. Place the oil in a large ovenproof nonstick skillet, over high heat, until the oil is almost smoking.

5. Place the cakes in the hot oil and cook over medium-high heat for about 3 minutes, until browned. Turn and cook for about 2 minutes. Place the pan in the hot oven and bake for another 9 to 10 minutes. Serve.

Thick-Cut Yam Fries

SERVINGS: 2 ▌ **SERVING SIZE:** ABOUT 1½ CUPS FRIES ▌ THIS RECIPE CAN EASILY BE MULTIPLIED ▌ **COOKING TIME:** 25 MINUTES

2 small yams (about 5 ounces each)
Spray olive oil
¼ teaspoon salt
Freshly ground black pepper
⅛ teaspoon dried thyme

NUTRITION FACTS

Serving size about 1½ cups fries
Servings 2
Calories 185
Calories from Fat 22
Total Fat 2 g (4%)
Saturated Fat <1g (2%)
Trans Fat 0 g
Monounsaturated Fat 2 g
Cholesterol 0 mg (0%)
Sodium 303 mg (13%)
Total Carbohydrates 39 g (13%)
Dietary Fiber 6 g (23%)
Sugars 1 g
Protein 2 g
Vitamin A (4%)
Vitamin C (40%)
Calcium (3%)
Iron (5%)

*Parenthetical percentages refer to % Daily Value.

Sweet potatoes are not true yams. What is marketed in the United States as a sweet potato is usually a potato with a pale skin and creamy yellow flesh. These are closely related to russet potatoes and are drier and not very sweet. What is usually sold as a yam is actually the darker-skinned sweet potato. The thick orange skin is tough and fibrous and the flesh is moist, with a rich orange color.

1. Place a large ovenproof skillet in the oven and preheat the oven to 325°F.

2. Scrub the yams well and then cut into wedges. It's easiest to cut them in half lengthwise and then quarters and then eighths.

3. When the oven is hot, spray the pan lightly with oil. Add the yam wedges and sprinkle the salt, pepper, and thyme over the top. Spray lightly with olive oil.

4. Return the pan to the oven and bake for about 25 minutes, tossing frequently. Serve hot.

Iceberg Salad with Blue Cheese Dressing

SERVINGS: 1 ▐ **SERVING SIZE:** 1 WEDGE SALAD ▐ THIS RECIPE CAN EASILY BE
MULTIPLIED ▐ **COOKING TIME:** 15 MINUTES

⅛ medium-size head iceberg
    lettuce
1 tablespoon candied
    pecans
2 tablespoons blue cheese
    dressing

NUTRITION FACTS

Serving size 1 wedge salad
Servings 1
Calories 75
Calories from Fat 26
Total Fat 3 g (5%)
Saturated Fat 2 g (8%)
Trans Fat 0 g
Monounsaturated Fat 1 g
Cholesterol 8 mg (3%)
Sodium 368 mg (15%)
Total Carbohydrates 9 g (3%)
Dietary Fiber 2 g (8%)
Sugars 6 g
Protein 4 g
Vitamin A (15%)
Vitamin C (7%)
Calcium (10%)
Iron (4%)

*Parenthetical percentages
refer to % Daily Value.

Blue cheeses are generally a medium fat cheese, having between 8 and 9 grams of fat per ounce. Some are higher in fat, with up to 12 grams per ounce, but as with so many flavorful cheeses, a little can go a long way. Blue cheeses contain a fair amount of sodium, so you may not have to add salt to recipes that use blue cheese.

Place the lettuce on a plate and top with the pecans and blue cheese dressing.

Roast Turkey Breast

SERVINGS: 8 ▮ SERVING SIZE: 4 OUNCES TURKEY BREAST ▮ COOKING TIME: 90 MINUTES

1 (3-pound) bone-in turkey breast
3 sprigs (about 3 tablespoons) fresh rosemary

NUTRITION FACTS

Serving size 4 ounces turkey breast
Servings 8
Calories 150
Calories from Fat 28
Total Fat 3 g (5%)
Saturated Fat 1 g (4%)
Trans Fat 0 g
Monounsaturated Fat 1 g
Cholesterol 88 mg (29%)
Sodium 52 mg (2%)
Total Carbohydrates 0 g (0%)
Dietary Fiber 0 g (0%)
Sugars 0 g
Protein 28 g
Vitamin A (0%)
Vitamin C (0%)
Calcium (1%)
Iron (9%)

*Parenthetical percentages refer to % Daily Value.

The nutrition information for this recipe includes the skin. Most nutritionists will tell you not to eat chicken or turkey skin, because that's where all the fat is. Dr. Gourmet recipes that use chicken or turkey generally follow this guideline, but I do feel that on holidays such as Thanksgiving, it's good to splurge. Being healthy day to day lets you feel better about yourself all year long, including on special days. Eat the skin if you like, because holidays are the time to splurge and roast turkey is the perfect comfort food to splurge on.

This recipe does makes great leftovers as sandwiches but also as Roasted Turkey, Wild Rice, and Cranberry Salad (page 281).

Serve with Mashed Yams or Cornbread Dressing and Roasted Acorn Squash or Roasted Beets or Herbed Zucchini.

1. Preheat the oven to 325°F.
2. Rinse the whole turkey breast in cold water and pat dry.
3. Starting at the peak of the turkey breast, pull back the skin and slide a finger between the skin and the turkey breast on either side of the peak of the breast bone. This will form a small pocket.
4. Insert half of the rosemary into each of the pockets, pushing it as far down as possible and working to distribute the rosemary leaves over the face of the breast meat, between the breast meat and the skin.

5. Place the turkey breast in a large roasting pan and place the pan in the preheated oven. Roast for 30 minutes, then turn the roasting pan 180° in the oven (to make sure the turkey roasts evenly). After 1 hour, cover the skin of the breast with aluminum foil. If the skin is not quite crispy, that's okay.

6. After 90 to 105 minutes, remove the aluminum foil and roast until the internal temperature of the breast meat is 160°F.

7. Transfer to a cutting board and allow to rest for at least 10 minutes before carving.

DAY 49 | DINNER

Roasted Acorn Squash

SERVINGS: 4 ▌ SERVING SIZE: ¼ SQUASH ▌ THIS RECIPE CAN BE EASILY MULTIPLIED ▌ THE LEFTOVERS MAKE A GOOD INGREDIENT IN TOSSED SALADS ▌ COOKING TIME: 30 MINUTES

1 acorn squash (about 1 pound)
2 teaspoons butter
2 teaspoons brown sugar

NUTRITION FACTS

Serving size ¼ squash
Servings 4
Calories 56
Calories from Fat 10
Total Fat 3 g (4%)
Saturated Fat 1 g (5%)
Trans Fats 0 g
Monounsaturated Fat 1 g
Cholesterol 3 mg (1%)
Sodium 4 mg (<1%)
Total Carbohydrates 13 g (4%)
Dietary Fiber 2 g (7%)
Sugars 1 g
Protein 1 g
Vitamin A (9%)
Vitamin C (20%)
Calcium (4%)
Iron (5%)

*Parenthetical percentages refer to % Daily Value.

Simple dishes are the best. Pair this roasted acorn squash with a roasted salmon dish such as the Salmon with Caper Mayonnaise (page 252) and you have the nearly perfect meal.

1. Preheat the oven to 400°F.

2. Halve the squash lengthwise. Scoop out the seeds and discard them. Make shallow cuts in a grid pattern along the inside of the squash.

3. Place 1 teaspoon of the butter and 1 teaspoon of the brown sugar in the cavity of each squash.

4. Set the squash, cavity side up, in the preheated oven and lower the heat to 350°F. Roast for about 30 minutes. Using a spoon, occasionally baste the top and inside of the squash with the butter mixture.

5. Remove and serve after allowing to cool for about 5 minutes.

Roasted Yams with Rosemary

SERVINGS: 4 ▌ **SERVING SIZE:** ABOUT 1 CUP ▌ THIS RECIPE CAN EASILY BE DOUBLED OR TRIPLED, USING A VERY LARGE PAN ▌ **COOKING TIME:** 25 MINUTES

1 tablespoon olive oil
1 medium-size white onion, diced
1½ pounds yams, peeled and cut into ½-inch cubes
¼ teaspoon salt
Freshly ground black pepper
1 tablespoon fresh rosemary, or 1 teaspoon dried

NUTRITION FACTS

Serving size 1 cup
Servings 4
Calories 246
Calories from Fat 33
Total Fat 4 g (6%)
Saturated Fat 1 g (3%)
Trans Fat 0 g
Monounsaturated Fat 2.5 g
Cholesterol 0 mg (0%)
Sodium 162 mg (7%)
Total Carbohydrates 51 g (17%)
Dietary Fiber 8 g (30%)
Sugars 2 g
Protein 3 g
Vitamin A (5%)
Vitamin C (52%)
Calcium (4%)
Iron (6%)

*Parenthetical percentages refer to % Daily Value.

This recipe is as good cold as it is hot (maybe better) and will keep in the refrigerator for about 48 hours.

1. Place a large ovenproof skillet in the oven and preheat the oven to 375°F.
2. When the oven is hot, place 1 teaspoon of the olive oil and the onion in the heated pan. Stir well and return the pan to the oven. Stir the onion about every 5 minutes.
3. After 10 minutes, add the yams and stir well. Increase the temperature of the oven to 375°F. Stir the yams every 5 to 7 minutes. It will take about 40 minutes for them to cook. About 10 minutes before the yams are done (when they have begun to soften), add the salt, pepper, and rosemary. The yams are done when they are tender but not mushy.
4. Remove from the oven and place in a large bowl. Stir in the remaining 2 teaspoons of olive oil and serve (or chill).

Steamed Clams with Spicy Tomato Corn Broth

SERVINGS: 2 ▌ **SERVING SIZE:** 12 CLAMS WITH 2 OUNCES PASTA ▌ THIS RECIPE CAN EASILY BE MULTIPLIED ▌ **COOKING TIME:** 30 MINUTES

4 ounces fettuccine noodles
1 teaspoon unsalted butter
¼ cup minced shallots
1 medium-size carrot, cut into small dice
1 small rib celery, cut into small dice
½ cup white wine
2 tablespoons tomato paste
⅛ teaspoon salt
⅛ teaspoon cayenne
24 littleneck clams
¼ cup corn kernels
1 slice prosciutto, cut into small dice
½ medium-size tomato, seeded and diced
2 tablespoons fresh flat-leaf parsley
2 (1-ounce) slices French or sourdough bread

NUTRITION FACTS

Serving size 12 clams with 2 ounces pasta
Servings 2
Calories 488
Calories from Fat 50
Total Fat 6 g (9%)
Saturated Fat 2 g (10%)
Trans Fats 0 g
Monounsaturated Fat 1 g
Cholesterol 50 mg (17%)
Sodium 760 mg (32%)
Total Carbohydrates 71 g (24%)
Dietary Fiber 5 g (18%)
Sugars 7 g
Protein 27 g
Vitamin A (136%)
Vitamin C (55%)
Calcium (12%)
Iron (108%)

*Parenthetical percentages refer to % Daily Value.

1. Place 3 quarts of water in a stockpot over high heat. When it boils, add the fettuccine and cook, stirring occasionally, until almost done. There should be a slight firmness to the pasta.

2. Drain, rinse, and set aside after dividing between two large soup bowls.

3. Heat the butter in a medium-size stockpot over medium-low heat. Add the shallots, carrot, and celery. Cook for about 2 minutes, until slightly soft. Add the white wine, tomato paste, salt, and cayenne, and ½ cup of water.

4. Increase the heat to high and, as the water begins to boil, stir to blend the tomato paste into the broth.

5. Add the clams, corn, and prosciutto. Cover and cook, stirring once or twice, until all of the clams have opened.

6. Using tongs, place half of the opened clams in each bowl on top of the pasta. Pour the broth over the clams and pasta. Top with the tomato and parsley.

7. Serve with the French bread.

Tamale Pie with Black Beans

SERVINGS: 6 ▌ SERVING SIZE: ABOUT 2 CUPS ▌ THIS RECIPE CAN EASILY BE DOUBLED
OR TRIPLED, USING SEPARATE PANS ▌ COOKING TIME: 45 MINUTES

1 teaspoon olive oil
2 cloves garlic, minced
1 (10-ounce) package frozen
    chopped onions
1 (10-ounce) package frozen
    mixed peppers
1 (15-ounce) can no-salt-
    added diced tomatoes
1 teaspoon ground cumin
½ teaspoon chili powder
½ teaspoon salt
2 (15-ounce) cans no-salt-
    added black beans,
    drained and rinsed
Spray cooking oil
8 taco shells
8 ounces reduced-fat
    Monterey Jack cheese

NUTRITION FACTS

Serving size about 2 cups
Servings 6
Calories 356
Calories from Fat 117
Total Fat 13 g   (20%)
Saturated Fat 6 g (31%)
Trans Fat 0 g
Monounsaturated Fat 5 g
Cholesterol 24 mg (8%)
Sodium 482 mg (20%)
Total Carbohydrates 41 g (14%)
Dietary Fiber 11 g (42%)
Sugars 5 g
Protein 21 g
Vitamin A (10%)
Vitamin C (78%)
Calcium (34%)
Iron (19%)

*Parenthetical percentages
refer to % Daily Value.

Growing up, this had a lot of names depending on whose house I was at—tortilla casserole, taco casserole, tamale pie, it didn't matter. And there are endless variations. This one was created to be as simple as possible and to use items out of your pantry or freezer.

This is also made to be more family friendly and is less spicy than some folks might want. A bit more cumin (an extra teaspoon) and chili powder (another ½ teaspoon) will give it more flavor. Adding a bit of cayenne will also help add the zing you might crave. Be sure to check the sodium and trans fat content of your taco shells.

This recipe keeps well as leftovers in the refrigerator.

1. Preheat the oven to 375°F.

2. Place the oil in a large skillet, over medium-high heat. Add the minced garlic while the pan is heating, stirring frequently.

3. When the pan is hot, add the onions and peppers. Cook for about 5 minutes, stirring frequently.

4. Add the tomatoes, cumin, chili powder, and salt and cook for 10 minutes. Stir occasionally.

5. Fold the beans into the tomato mixture.

6. Lightly coat a 10-inch oblong pan with the cooking spray. Add one-third of the tomato mixture to the bottom of the pan. Top with a layer of four of the taco shells broken in half to lie flat.

7. Add another third of the tomato mixture on top of the taco shells. Top this with one-third of the cheese. Top with a layer of four of the taco shells broken in half to lie flat.

8. Add the final third of the tomato bean mixture on top of the taco shells. Top this with the remaining cheese.

9. Bake in the preheated oven for 15 minutes.

DAY 52 | DINNER

Mojo Pork Tenderloin

SERVINGS: 4 ▌ SERVING SIZE: 4 OUNCES PORK ▌ THIS RECIPE CAN EASILY BE HALVED OR MULTIPLIED ▌ COOKING TIME: 60 MINUTES

Juice of 2 navel oranges
Juice of 1 lime
¼ cup flat-leaf parsley, chopped finely
1 tablespoon fresh oregano, chopped finely
1 teaspoon fresh thyme
1 cloves garlic, minced
¼ teaspoon salt
1 tablespoon extra-virgin olive oil
16 ounces (1 large) pork tenderloin, well trimmed

Dollar for dollar, this is one of the best cuts of meat going. Pork tenderloin is lean and flavorful. You can roast it, braise it, grill it, or cut it into medallions—almost anything. This recipe can be doubled for two tenderloins, since in most grocery stores they are sold in two-packs, each tenderloin in the pack being about a pound. Ask the butcher if you want only one.

There will be a variable amount of fat and I trim this carefully. Most important is the silverskin. This is a thin layer of fascia at the head of the tenderloin on one side. It has to be trimmed because it is tough and fibrous. Lay the tenderloin on the cutting board, silverskin side up. Press gently to flatten the meat. Slip the point of your filet knife under the fascia and cut toward the end of the tenderloin. Keep the pressure slightly upward and the silverskin will easily cut away from the meat.

Leftovers are great for sandwiches.

[CONTINUES]

1. Mix together the orange juice, lime juice, parsley, oregano, thyme, garlic, salt, and olive oil in a large glass bowl. (This makes approximately 3 cups.)

2. Place the pork tenderloin in a zippered plastic bag and add 2 cups of the marinade. Seal the bag and marinate at least overnight. Place the remaining marinade in the refrigerator.

3. When you are ready to cook the pork, place a large nonstick skillet in the oven and preheat to 375°F.

4. While the pan is preheating, strain the cup of extra marinade and discard the herbs and garlic. Place the strained marinade in a small saucepan over high heat and bring to a boil. Lower the heat to medium and simmer gently to reduce by half.

5. Remove the pork tenderloins from the bag and place them on a plate. Strain the remaining marinade from the bag, reserving the liquid to use for basting.

6. Place the pork tenderloins in the preheated pan and return the pan to the oven. Cook for about 4 minutes and turn, then turn the pork every 3 minutes after that, until all the sides are seared. After the second turn, baste with ½ cup of the marinade, coating the tenderloin well. While cooking, stir the reducing sauce.

7. As the pork cooks and the marinade is reduced, continue to baste with ¼ to ½ cup at a time to create a caramelized glaze on the pork. It should take 20 to 25 minutes to reach an internal temperature of 160°F. As the pork is finishing, add the remaining marinade to the pan to create a syrupy sauce.

8. Remove the pork from the oven and let rest on the counter for about 3 minutes before carving. Serve topped with the reduced sauce from the pan.

Coconut Rice

SERVINGS: 2 ▌ **SERVING SIZE:** ½ CUP COOKED RICE ▌ THIS RECIPE CAN EASILY BE MULTIPLIED BY 2, 3, OR 4 ▌ **COOKING TIME:** 25 MINUTES

½ cup reduced-fat (light) unsweetened coconut milk
¼ teaspoon salt
½ cup uncooked jasmine rice

NUTRITION FACTS

Serving size about ½ cup cooked rice
Servings 2
Calories 211
Calories from Fat 35
Total Fat 4 g (6%)
Saturated Fat 3 g (14%)
Trans Fats 0 g
Monounsaturated Fat 0 g
Cholesterol 0 mg (0%)
Sodium 304 mg (13%)
Total Carbohydrates 38 g (13%)
Dietary Fiber 1 g (2%)
Sugars 1 g
Protein 3 g
Vitamin A (0%)
Vitamin C (0%)
Calcium (2%)
Iron (12%)

*Parenthetical percentages refer to % Daily Value.

The canned coconut milk used in this recipe is a reduced-fat version. This will sometimes be labeled "light" or "lite" coconut milk. There is a big difference between regular coconut milk, at 45 grams of fat per cup, and the light version, at about 12 grams of fat per cup. In both regular and light coconut milk, most of the fat is highly saturated, so I always try to use coconut milk sparingly.

1. Prior to opening the can of coconut milk, shake very well.

2. In a medium-size saucepan, heat the coconut milk, ¾ cup of water, and salt. When the liquid boils, stir in the jasmine rice.

3. Lower the heat to medium-low and simmer, covered, for about 15 minutes. Do not boil away all of the liquid and do not stir the rice.

4. When a very small amount of liquid remains, remove the pan from the burner and let it stand, covered, for 5 minutes before serving.

Roasted Beets

SERVINGS: 2 ▌ **SERVING SIZE:** ABOUT 1 CUP BEETS ▌ THIS RECIPE CAN EASILY BE MULTIPLIED BY 2, 3, OR 4, BUT A LARGER ROASTING PAN MUST BE USED ▌ **COOKING TIME:** 45 MINUTES

2 medium-size beets
1 teaspoon unsalted butter
¼ teaspoon salt
⅛ teaspoon dried oregano
⅛ teaspoon chili powder

NUTRITION FACTS

Serving size 1 cup
Servings 2
Calories 44
Calories from Fat 10
Total Fat 1 g (2%)
Saturated Fat 1 g (3%)
Trans Fats 0 g
Monounsaturated Fat 0 g
Cholesterol 2 mg (1%)
Sodium 210 mg (9%)
Total Carbohydrates 8 g (3%)
Dietary Fiber 2 g (9%)
Sugars 6 g
Protein 1 g
Vitamin A (2%)
Vitamin C (7%)
Calcium (1%)
Iron (4%)

*Parenthetical percentages refer to % Daily Value.

These are the veggies that you probably hated as a kid (I did). Most of us had them out of a can or as pickled beets, but fresh beets are fantastic and nothing like canned.

Look for fresh beets with the beet greens still attached. The greens should be fresh and crisp, like fresh spinach. The greens are delicious sautéed quickly in just a pat of butter and a touch of maple syrup (like the Collard Greens, page 41). They should be cooked as soon as possible because they will wilt rapidly.

You are not stuck with red beets—there are also white, yellow, golden, and striped beets. Golden beets are milder than red, but they are still very sweet. The bonus is that they don't bleed like red beets. Striped beets have rings of red and white stripes. They are also known as Chiogga (kee oh ja) beets.

Leftovers are great ingredients in tossed salads.

1. Preheat the oven to 400°F.
2. Wrap the beets in a paper towel and cook on HIGH in the microwave for 5 minutes. Let cool for 5 minutes.
3. Peel and cut into 1-inch cubes. Place in a roasting pan large enough so that the beets are not completely touching.
4. Put the pat of butter on the beets and sprinkle the salt, oregano, and chili powder over the top.
5. Lower the heat to 375°F and roast for 20 to 25 minutes. The beets are done when they are slightly crisp on the outside.

Roasted Turkey, Wild Rice, and Cranberry Salad

SERVINGS: 6 ▎ **SERVING SIZE:** ABOUT 2 CUPS ▎ THIS RECIPE CAN EASILY BE DOUBLED ▎
COOKING TIME: 30 MINUTES

½ plus ¼ teaspoon salt
1 cup uncooked wild rice
¼ teaspoon dried rosemary
⅓ cup dried sweetened
    cranberries
¼ cup chopped pecans
1 small shallot, minced
2 ribs celery, diced
¼ red bell pepper, seeded
    and diced
12 ounces roasted turkey
    breast, cut into ½-inch
    cubes
½ cup reduced-fat
    mayonnaise

NUTRITION FACTS

Serving size 2 cups
Servings 6
Calories 281
Calories from Fat 93
Total Fat 11 g (16%)
Saturated Fat 1 g (7%)
Trans Fat 0 g
Monounsaturated Fat 2 g
Cholesterol 42 mg (14%)
Sodium 491 mg (20%)
Total Carbohydrates 29 g (10%)
Dietary Fiber 3 g (11%)
Sugars 7 g
Protein 19 g
Vitamin A (6%)
Vitamin C (14%)
Calcium (2%)
Iron (8%)

*Parenthetical percentages
refer to % Daily Value.

While this is perfect for that leftover holiday turkey, it's a fantastic recipe that you can make with almost any meat. Try leftover roasted chicken breast, flank steak, or pork tenderloin. Even though it's a chilled salad, its hearty ingredients make it a great part of a cold-weather meal.

This recipe makes great leftovers.

1. In a medium-size saucepan, heat 3 cups of water and ½ teaspoon of the salt. When the water boils, stir in the wild rice.

2. Lower the heat to medium-low and simmer, partially covered, for about 15 minutes. Do not boil away all of the liquid and do not stir the rice.

3. When a very small amount of liquid remains, remove the pan from the burner and let it stand, covered, for 5 minutes. Remove from the saucepan and place in a large mixing bowl. Let cool for about 10 minutes and then put in the refrigerator for 15 minutes to cool.

4. When the rice is cool add the rosemary, cranberries, pecans, shallot, celery, red pepper, turkey breast, mayonnaise, and remaining ¼ teaspoon of salt to the bowl and fold together gently. Chill for at least 40 minutes.

Fusilli with Smoked Gouda and Chicken

SERVINGS: 4 ▌ SERVING SIZE: ABOUT 2 CUPS ▌ THIS RECIPE CAN EASILY BE MULTIPLIED
▌ COOKING TIME: 30 MINUTES

1 cooked rotisserie chicken
8 ounces whole wheat fusilli
1 teaspoon olive oil
1 onion, diced
2 cloves garlic, minced
1 red bell pepper, seeded
    and cut into large dice
2 (15-ounce) cans diced
    tomatoes
1 teaspoon dried thyme
1 teaspoon dried marjoram
Freshly ground black
    pepper
4 ounces smoked Gouda
    cheese, shredded
1 ounce Parmigiano-
    Reggiano, grated

NUTRITION FACTS

Serving size about 2 cups
Servings 4
Calories 531
Calories from Fat 154
Total Fat 17 g (27%)
Saturated Fat 8 g (40%)
Trans Fat 0 g
Monounsaturated Fat 6 g
Cholesterol 100 mg (33%)
Sodium 551 mg (19%)
Total Carbohydrates 56 g
    (23%)
Dietary Fiber 8 g (32%)
Sugars 3 g
Protein 41 g
Vitamin A (39%)
Vitamin C (88%)
Calcium (37%)
Iron (29%)

*Parenthetical percentages
refer to % Daily Value.

Using a precooked rotisserie chicken from the grocery can really speed up your meals. This is a great comfort food recipe that takes advantage of someone else's cooking the chicken for you. Most of the time, the cooked chickens are not any more expensive than the uncooked.

While the water is coming to a boil you can easily skin and debone the chicken. The rest of the assembly takes about 10 minutes and the result is a warm, comforting, and still elegant pasta bake.

This recipe makes great leftovers.

1. Place 3 quarts of water in a large stockpot over high heat.
2. While the water is coming to a boil, remove and discard the skin of the chicken. Remove all the meat and tear into medium-size shreds.
3. When the water boils, add the fusilli. Cook for about 10 minutes until it is al dente. The pasta should be just slightly underdone. Drain the pasta.
4. Preheat the oven to 325°F.
5. Place the olive oil in a large skillet over medium heat. Add the onions and garlic and cook for about 5 minutes, stirring frequently. Add the bell pepper and cook for another 3 to 4 minutes.
6. Add the tomatoes, thyme, marjoram, and ground pepper. Stir well.
7. Add the shredded chicken and stir well. Add the pasta and stir until blended. Add the shredded Gouda and stir well.

8. Place the pasta in a 10-inch oblong Pyrex dish. Place in the oven and bake for about 15 minutes. Sprinkle the Parmesan over the top and bake for another 2 minutes. Serve.

DAY 55 | DINNER

Indian Shrimp Curry

SERVINGS: 4 ▌ SERVING SIZE: ABOUT 2 CUPS (4 OUNCES SHRIMP) ▌ THIS RECIPE CAN EASILY BE MULTIPLIED ▌ COOKING TIME: 30 MINUTES

2 teaspoons extra-virgin olive oil
2 cloves garlic, minced
1 medium-size white onion, sliced
1 medium-size red onion, sliced
1 tablespoon cornstarch
1 cup 2% milk
1 tablespoon curry powder
2 tablespoons honey
½ teaspoon salt
1 cup low-fat (light) unsweet-ened coconut milk
1 pound large shrimp, peeled and deveined
4 tablespoons fresh cilantro leaves

NUTRITION FACTS

Serving size about 2 cups (jasmine rice not included)
Servings 4
Calories 272
Calories from Fat 84
Total Fat 10 g (15%)
Saturated Fat 5 g (25%)
Trans Fats 0 g
Monounsaturated Fat 3 g
Cholesterol 175 mg (58%)
Sodium 499 mg (21%)
Total Carbohydrates 20 g (7%)
Dietary Fiber 1 g (5%)
Sugars 14 g
Protein 26 g
Vitamin A (6%)
Vitamin C (12%)
Calcium (17%)
Iron (22%)

*Parenthetical percentages refer to % Daily Value.

Serve with Coconut Rice (page 279).

Leftovers are great. Reheat gently.

1. Heat the olive oil in large nonstick skillet over medium-high heat.

2. Add the garlic and white and red onions and lower the heat to medium. Cook gently, stirring frequently, until the onions begin to soften.

3. While the onions are cooking, place the cornstarch in a cup and add ¼ cup of the milk, stirring until the cornstarch is dissolved.

4. After the onions are soft, add the curry powder, honey, salt, coconut milk, and the remaining milk to the skillet. Stir well until the ingredients are well blended, then add the cornstarch mixture.

5. Lower the heat to medium-low and cook for about 3 minutes.

6. Add the shrimp and simmer until they are opaque in center, about 5 minutes.

7. Serve the curry over jasmine rice and top with 1 tablespoon of cilantro leaves per serving.

Orzo with Dill Pesto and Halibut

SERVINGS: 2 ▌ SERVING SIZE: ABOUT 1 CUP OF PASTA WITH VEGGIES AND FISH ▌ THIS
RECIPE CAN EASILY BE MULTIPLIED ▌ COOKING TIME: 30 MINUTES

4 ounces orzo
Spray olive oil
1 medium-size zucchini, cut
    into ½-inch-thick
    rounds
8 ounces halibut fillet
12 (6 ounces) grape
    tomatoes
1 tablespoon pine nuts
1 ounce goat cheese
3 tablespoons dill pesto
    (recipe follows)
¼ teaspoon salt
Freshly ground black
    pepper

NUTRITION FACTS

Serving size about 1 cup of
    pasta with veggies and fish
Servings 2
Calories 524
Calories from Fat 159
Total Fat 18 g (28%)
Saturated Fat 4 g (21%)
Trans Fats 0 g
Monounsaturated Fat 6 g
Cholesterol 45 mg (15%)
Sodium 476 mg (20%)
Total Carbohydrates 52 g (17%)
Dietary Fiber 5 g (19%)
Sugars 6 g
Protein 38 g
Vitamin A (21%)
Vitamin C (59%)
Calcium (18%)
Iron (29%)

*Parenthetical percentages
refer to % Daily Value.

This is another of a series of dishes designed as much for use as leftovers as for serving right away. The key is to slightly undercook the fish and then microwave the leftovers very gently. Heat for about 90 seconds on HIGH *and then remove and stir. Repeat. It will take between 4 and 6 minutes to reheat, depending on your microwave. This recipe will keep well for about 72 hours in the fridge.*

1. Place a large ovenproof skillet in the oven and preheat the oven to 425°F.

2. Place 3 quarts of water in a large saucepan over high heat. When the water is boiling, add the orzo. Lower the heat to medium-high so the water won't boil over.

3. While the pasta is cooking, spray the hot pan lightly with olive oil and place the sliced zucchini and the halibut in the pan. Return the pan to the oven.

4. The pasta will take 10 to 13 minutes to cook. The fish will not take as long and should be turned after about 5 minutes. At 10 minutes, remove the fish from the pan, turn the zucchini over, and return the pan to the oven.

5. When the pasta is done, strain it and return the pasta to the saucepan. Add the tomatoes, pine nuts, goat cheese, dill pesto, salt, and pepper. Stir until the goat cheese is melted and the dill pesto is well blended.

6. Gently flake the cooked fish into the saucepan and fold it into the orzo. Serve, topped with the cooked zucchini.

7. If you are making it to be used later, divide the orzo and halibut mixture between two plastic containers and top with the cooked zucchini. Let cool for about 20 minutes, cover, and refrigerate.

DAY 56 | DINNER

Dill Pesto

SERVINGS: 6 ▮ SERVING SIZE: 2 TABLESPOONS ▮ THIS RECIPE CAN EASILY BE DOUBLED ▮ COOKING TIME: 15 MINUTES ▮ THIS DILL PESTO KEEPS WELL FOR UP TO A WEEK IN THE REFRIGERATOR

2 tablespoons pine nuts
2 cloves garlic, minced
4 cups fresh dill
1 ounce Parmigiano-Reggiano, grated
2 teaspoons fresh lemon juice
2 tablespoons extra-virgin olive oil

Combine the pine nuts, garlic, fresh dill, Parmesan, lemon juice, olive oil, and 2 tablespoons of water in a blender and blend until smooth. Chill thoroughly.

NUTRITION FACTS

Serving size 2 tablespoons
Servings 6
Calories 92
Calories from Fat 76
Total Fat 9 g (14%)
Saturated Fat 2 g (8%)
Trans Fat 0 g
Monounsaturated Fat 5 g
Cholesterol 3 mg (1%)
Sodium 76 mg (3%)
Total Carbohydrates 1 g (<1%)
Dietary Fiber 0 g (1%)
Sugars 0 g
Protein 2 g
Vitamin A (9%)
Vitamin C (9%)
Calcium (7%)
Iron (4%)

*Parenthetical percentages refer to % Daily Value.

Chocolate Cheesecake

SERVINGS: 12 ▎ **SERVING SIZE:** $\frac{1}{12}$ CAKE ▎ **COOKING TIME:** 60 MINUTES ▎ KEEPS 48 TO 60 HOURS, TIGHTLY COVERED

CRUST
10 Nabisco Famous Chocolate Wafers
8 squares low-fat graham crackers
2 tablespoons Dutch-processed cocoa powder
2 tablespoons Splenda
1 tablespoon canola oil

FILLING
2 tablespoons instant coffee granules
3.5 ounces bittersweet baking chocolate
1 (8-ounce) block nonfat cream cheese
1 (8-ounce) block reduced-fat cream cheese
1 cup 1% cottage cheese
1 cup nonfat sour cream
1½ cups Splenda
¾ cup Dutch-processed cocoa powder
1 (4-ounce) carton egg substitute
½ teaspoon pure vanilla extract
½ teaspoon salt
3 egg whites

I do love cheesecake and this chocolate version is a great dessert. It hits all the right notes with creamy chocolate but is only a little more than 200 calories per serving.

1. This recipe requires a 9-inch springform pan and 18-inch wide aluminum foil. Remove the sides from the springform pan and place the bottom of the pan on top of two 18-inch square sheets of aluminum foil. Fold the edges of the foil into a loose cone shape so that the sides of the pan can be slipped down over the top. Close the sides of the pan and then press the foil against the inside of the pan. The end result will be the foil outside the pan on the bottom and inside the pan on the sides.

2. Fill a large roasting pan (large enough to fit the springform pan into without its touching the sides) with about 1½ inches of water and place in the oven. Preheat the oven to 300°F.

3. While the water bath is heating, prepare the crust. Place the chocolate wafers, graham crackers, cocoa powder, and Splenda in a food processor and process until they are fine crumbs. Slowly drizzle in the canola oil until it is well blended into the crumbs. Place the crumb mixture in the springform pan and gently press the crumbs into the bottom of the pan.

4. Prepare the filling. Place the coffee granules and 2 tablespoons of water in a double boiler over high heat (or a Pyrex bowl set over a pot of boiling water). Add the baking chocolate and stir while it melts slowly.

5. When the chocolate sauce is smooth, remove from the heat and place in a food processor bowl fitted with a steel blade. Add the cheese and sour cream, Splenda, cocoa powder, egg substitute, vanilla extract, and salt. Process until smooth.

6. In a copper bowl, whisk the egg whites until they form stiff peaks. Gently fold the batter from the food processor into the egg whites until well blended.

7. Pour the batter into the springform pan. Place the pan in the water bath and cook for 1 hour. Turn off the oven and remove the water bath. Return the cheesecake to the oven and allow it to sit for 2 hours in the oven as it cools.

8. Chill for at least 4 hours before serving. Serve with a fork and a smile.

Crème Caramel (Flan)

¼ cup sugar
1 (4-ounce) carton egg
    substitute
2 large egg yolks
½ cup Z-sweet stevia
1 tablespoon pure vanilla
    extract
2 cups 1% milk

NUTRITION FACTS

Serving size 1 flan
Servings 6
Calories 125
Calories from Fat 28
Total Fat 3 g (5%)
Saturated Fat 1 g (6%)
Trans Fats 0 g
Monounsaturated Fat 1 g
Cholesterol 74 mg (24%)
Sodium 84 mg (3%)
Total Carbohydrates 17 g (6%)
Dietary Fiber <1 g (0%)
Sugars 12 g
Protein 6 g
Vitamin A (6%)
Vitamin C (2%)
Calcium (13%)
Iron (3%)

This is the perfect dessert for your dinner party: rich, creamy, and only 125 calories. Your guests will love you for it.

1. Place the sugar and ½ cup of water in a saucepan and stir until the sugar dissolves. Slowly heat over high heat until the syrup boils. Allow it to boil until it begins to brown. Swirl the pan only if the caramel appears to be browning unevenly.

2. Divide the caramel among six individual ramekins.

3. Preheat the oven to 325°F.

4. In a separate bowl, whisk together the egg substitute, egg yolks, stevia, and vanilla until smooth.

5. Place 2 quarts of water in a separate saucepan or teapot over high heat.

6. Place the milk in a saucepan over medium-high heat and bring to a boil, whisking frequently. The moment the milk begins to boil, remove it from the heat and slowly drizzle into the egg mixture, whisking continuously.

7. When all of the milk is well blended into the egg mixture, ladle the custard into the ramekins. Place the filled ramekins in a shallow roasting pan. Fill the pan with hot water until it is about halfway up the sides of the ramekins.

8. Place the water bath with the ramekins in the preheated oven and cook for 35 minutes.

9. Remove the custards from the water bath and allow them to cool. Cover with plastic wrap and chill in the refrigerator for at least 4 hours.

10. To serve, gently run a knife around the outer edge of the caramel. Place a plate upside down on top of each ramekin and invert the flan onto the plate.

Ice-Cream Sandwiches

SERVINGS: 1 ▊ **SERVING SIZE:** 2 ICE-CREAM SANDWICHES ▊ THIS RECIPE CAN EASILY BE MULTIPLIED ▊ **COOKING TIME:** 15 MINUTES

¼ cup light ice cream (100 calories per ½ cup)
4 Nabisco Famous Chocolate Wafers

NUTRITION FACTS

Serving size 2 ice-cream sandwiches
Servings 1
Calories 159
Calories from Fat 44
Total Fat 5 g (8%)
Saturated Fat 2 g (10%)
Trans Fat 0 g
Monounsaturated Fat 1 g
Cholesterol 6 mg (2%)
Sodium 163 mg (7%)
Total Carbohydrates 26 g (9%)
Dietary Fiber 1 g (4%)
Sugars 15 g
Protein 3 g
Vitamin A (3%)
Vitamin C (1%)
Calcium (6%)
Iron (5%)

*Parenthetical percentages refer to % Daily Value.

Simple and quick, these ice-cream sandwiches are a fun dessert for a treat or your next cookout.

1. Remove the ice cream from the freezer and let stand for about 10 minutes, until slightly soft.

2. Using a small ice-cream scoop, place about 2 tablespoons of ice cream on a chocolate wafer. Top with a second wafer and press together gently. Repeat. The sandwiches can be made and placed in the freezer for about 30 minutes.

Strawberry Shortcake

SERVINGS: 4 ▮ SERVING SIZE: 1 SLICE CAKE ▮ THIS RECIPE CAN EASILY BE DOUBLED OR TRIPLED ▮ COOKING TIME: 30 MINUTES

12 ounces strawberries, stemmed and sliced
2 teaspoons sugar
½ commercially prepared angel food cake
1 cup Strawberry Sauce (recipe follows)
12 tablespoons canned whipped cream

NUTRITION FACTS

Serving size 1 cup
Servings 4
Calories 179
Calories from Fat 23
Total Fat 3 g (4%)
Saturated Fat 1 g (7%)
Trans Fat 0 g
Monounsaturated Fat 1 g
Cholesterol 7 mg (2%)
Sodium 327 mg (14%)
Total Carbohydrates 37 g (12%)
Dietary Fiber 3 g (11%)
Sugars 9 g
Protein 4 g
Vitamin A (2%)
Vitamin C (110%)
Calcium (9%)
Iron (4%)

*Parenthetical percentages refer to % Daily Value.

Angel food cake is a great substitute for making your own shortcake and has fewer calories and less fat. The best part is that you don't have to spend time baking the shortcake. This is one place where I don't feel making it from scratch is necessary. The store-bought angel food cake is pretty darn good and most are made fresh on premises the morning you buy them. Although angel food cake keeps pretty well in the freezer, the result is less fluffy (but it is a little more like the texture of shortbread).

All of this, including the sauces, can be made the day before for a dinner party and is so simple but elegant, and a great dessert at under 200 calories. The Chocolate Strawberry Sauce adds a new twist to this comfort food recipe, but it's well worth the added 25 calories (you'll want to lick the plate).

This recipe requires the strawberry sauce to be made first. The strawberries will be good the next day.

1. Combine the sliced strawberries with the sugar. Toss well to coat the berries and place in the refrigerator for at least an hour.

2. Slice the half angel food cake into quarters. Cut each quarter in half for every serving you will need. Place the remaining cake in zippered plastic bags and put in the freezer.

3. When ready to serve, place ¼ cup of sauce on a plate and top with the sliced angel food cake. Top with one-quarter of the strawberry mixture and then 3 tablespoons of whipped cream.

Strawberry Sauce

SERVINGS: 4 ▌ SERVING SIZE: ABOUT ¼ CUP ▌ THIS RECIPE CAN EASILY BE DOUBLED OR TRIPLED ▌ COOKING TIME: 30 MINUTES ▌ KEEPS WELL IN THE REFRIGERATOR FOR 2 TO 3 DAYS

4 ounces fresh strawberries, stemmed and sliced

1 teaspoon sugar

NUTRITION FACTS

Serving size ¼ cup
Servings 4
Calories 13
Calories from Fat 1
Total Fat 0 g (0%)
Saturated Fat 0 g (0%)
Trans Fat 0 g
Monounsaturated Fat 0 g
Cholesterol 0 mg (0%)
Sodium 0 mg (0%)
Total Carbohydrates 3 g (1%)
Dietary Fiber 0 g (0%)
Sugars 2 g
Protein 0 g
Vitamin A (0%)
Vitamin C (0%)
Calcium (0%)
Iron (1%)

*Parenthetical percentages refer to % Daily Value.

Simple, straightforward. The best sauces don't require hours of time in the kitchen or dozens of ingredients. This sauce is fantastic over a scoop of ice cream or even as a topping for fruit. It is perfect for the Quick Strawberry Shortcake recipe, though.

1. Place the strawberries, 1 cup of water, and the sugar in a small stainless-steel or other nonreactive saucepan over medium heat. Simmer for 20 minutes.

2. Remove from the heat and let cool slightly. Puree, using a blender or stick blender.

3. Pass the sauce through a fine-mesh sieve. Chill the sauce for at least 1 hour before serving.

FOOD DIARY

WEEK / DAY	
DATE: TIME:	BREAKFAST/LUNCH/DINNER/SNACK:

WHAT	
HOW MUCH	
WHERE	
ACTIVITY	
MOOD	

NOTES

Introduction

1. Katherine Esposito, MD, PhD, et al., "Effects of a Mediterranean-Style Diet on the Need for Antihyperglycemic Drug Therapy in Patients with Newly Diagnosed Type 2 Diabetes: A Randomized Trial," *Annals of Internal Medicine* 151 (2009): 306–14.

2. As Dr. Brenda Davy reported at the meeting of the American Chemical Society, August 23, 2010.

Chapter 1: Week 1 Goals

1. David G. Schlundt, "The Role of Breakfast in the Treatment of Obesity: A Randomized Clinical Trial," *American Journal of Clinical Nutrition* 55 (1992): 645–51.

2. Sungsoo Cho, PhD, et al., "The Effect of Breakfast Type on Total Daily Energy Intake and Body Mass Index: Results from the Third National Health and Nutrition Examination Survey (NHANES III)," *Journal of the American College of Nutrition* 22 (2003): 296–302.

3. Rania Abou Samra and G. Harvey Anderson, "Insoluble Cereal Fiber Reduces Appetite and Short-Term Food Intake and Glycemic Response to Food Consumed 75 Min Later by Healthy Men," *American Journal of Clinical Nutrition* 86 (2007): 972–79.

4. Luc Djoussé, MD, MPH, DSc, et al., "Breakfast Cereals and Risk of Heart Failure in the Physicians' Health Study I," *Archives of Internal Medicine* 167 (2007): 2080–85.

5. Hamid R. Farshchi et al., "Deleterious Effects of Omitting Breakfast on Insulin Sensitivity and Fasting Lipid Profiles in Healthy Lean Women," *American Journal of Clinical Nutrition* 81 (2005): 388–96.

6. Karin Ried et al., "Effect of Garlic on Blood Pressure: A Systematic Review and Meta-Analysis," *BMC Cardiovascular Disorders* 8 (2008):13.

7. William E. Connor, "Will the Dietary Intake of Fish Prevent Atherosclerosis in Diabetic Women?" *American Journal of Clinical Nutrition* 80 (2004): 626–32.

8. Lydia A. Bazzano, PhD, et al., "Legume Consumption and Risk of Coronary Heart Disease in U.S. Men and Women," NHANES I Epidemiologic Follow-up Study *Archives of Internal Medicine* 161 (2001): 2573–78.

9. J. O. Prochaska and C. C. DiClemente, *The Transtheoretical Approach: Crossing Traditional Boundaries of Therapy* (Homewood, IL: Dow Jones–Irwin, 1984).

10. Bethany Ann Yon, MS, et al., "The Use of a Personal Digital Assistant for Dietary Self-Monitoring Does Not Improve the Validity of Self-Reports of Energy Intake," *Journal of the American Dietetic Association* 106 (2006): 1256–59.

11. Laura P. Svetkey, MD, et al., "Comparison of Strategies for Sustaining Weight Loss: The Weight Loss Maintenance Randomized Controlled Trial," *Journal of the American Medical Association* 299, no. 10 (2008): 1139–48.

12. Lydia Zepeda and David Deal, "Think Before You Eat: Photographic Food Diaries as Intervention Tools to Change Dietary Decision Making and Attitudes," *International Journal of Consumer Studies* 32 (2008): 692–98.

13. Jack F. Hollis et al., "Weight Loss During the Intensive Intervention Phase of the Weight-Loss Maintenance Trial," *American Journal of Preventative Medicine* 35, no. 2 (2008): 118–26.

14. Jeffrey J. VanWormer et al., "The Impact of Regular Self-Weighing on Weight Management: A Systematic Literature Review," *International Journal of Behavioral Nutrition and Physical Activity* 5 (2008): 54.

Chapter 2: Week 2 Goals

1. Frank M. Sacks, MD, et al., "Comparison of Weight-Loss Diets with Different Compositions of Fat, Protein, and Carbohydrates," *New England Journal of Medicine* 360 (2009): 859–73.

2. Ramon Estruch, MD, et al., "Effects of a Mediterranean-Style Diet on Cardiovascular Risk Factors: A Randomized Trial," *Annals of Internal Medicine* 145 (2006): 1–11.

3. Martha Clare Morris, ScD, et al., "Dietary Fats and the Risk of Incident Alzheimer Disease," *Archives of Neurology* 60 (2003): 194–200.

4. Jorge E. Chavarro, "Dietary Fatty Acid Intakes and the Risk of Ovulatory Infertility," *American Journal of Clinical Nutrition* 85 (2007): 231–37.

5. M. Macht and D. Dettmer, "Everyday Mood and Emotions After Eating a Chocolate Bar or an Apple," *Appetite* 46 (2006): 332–36.

6. P. K. Newby et al., "Intake of Whole Grains, Refined Grains, and Cereal Fiber Measured with 7-d Diet Records and Associations with Risk Factors for Chronic Disease," *American Journal of Clinical Nutrition* 86 (2007): 1745–53.

7. M. Bes-Rastrollo et al., "Association of Fiber Intake and Fruit/Vegetable Consumption with Weight Gain in a Mediterranean Population," *Nutrition* 22 (2006): 504–11.

8. Dariush Mozaffarian, MD, MPH, et al., "Cereal, Fruit, and Vegetable Fiber Intake and the Risk of Cardiovascular Disease in Elderly Individuals," *Journal of the American Medical Association* 289 (2003): 1659–66.

Chapter 3: Week 3 Goals

1. G. MacGregor and H. de Wardener, "Commentary: Salt, Blood Pressure and Health," *International Journal of Epidemiology* 31 (2002): 320–27.

2. INTERSALT Cooperative Research Group: "Findings of the International Cooperative INTERSALT study," *Hypertension* 17, suppl. I (1991): 9–15.

3. M. Bertino et al., "Long-Term Reduction in Dietary Sodium Alters the Taste of Salt," *American Journal of Clinical Nutrition* 36 (1982): 1134–44.

4. Lorraine T. Miller, PhD and Suk Y. Oh, PhD, "Effect of Dietary Egg on Variability of Plasma Cholesterol Levels and Lipoprotein Cholesterol," *American Journal of Clinical Nutrition* 42 (1985): 421–31.

5. Frank B. Hu, MD, et al., "A Prospective Study of Egg Consumption and Risk of Cardio-vascular Disease in Men and Women," *Journal of the American Medical Association* 281, no. 5 (1999): 1387–94.

6. J. S. Vander Wal et al., "Egg Breakfast Enhances Weight Loss," *International Journal of Obesity* 32 (2008): 1545–51.

7. Luc Djoussé, MD, MPH, DSc, "Egg Consumption and Risk of Heart Failure in the Physicians' Health Study," *Circulation* 117 (2008): 512–16.

8. Jaime Schwartz, MS, RD, "Portion Distortion: Typical Portion Sizes Selected by Young Adults," *Journal of the American Dietetic Association* 106 (2006): 1412–18.

9. Brian Wansink and Pierre Chandon, "Meal Size, Not Body Size, Explains Errors in Estimating the Calorie Content of Meals," *Annals of Internal Medicine* 145 (2006): 326–32.

10. Judy Kruger et al., "Dietary and Physical Activity Behaviors Among Adults Successful at Weight Loss Maintenance," *International Journal of Behavioral Nutrition and Physical Activity* 3:17 (2006): 3–17.

11. Jennifer O. Fisher et al., "Effects of Portion Size and Energy Density on Young Children's Intake at a Meal," *American Journal of Clinical Nutrition* 86 (2007): 174–79.

12. Brian Wansink et al., "Ice Cream Illusions: Bowls, Spoons, and Self-Served Portion Sizes," *American Journal of Preventative Medicine* 31 (2006): 240–43.

13. Sue D. Pedersen, MD, FRCPC, et al., "Portion Control Plate for Weight Loss in Obese Patients with Type 2 Diabetes Mellitus: A Controlled Clinical Trial," *Archives of Internal Medicine* 167 (2007): 1277–83.

Chapter 4: Week 4 Goals

1. Antonia Trichopoulou, MD, et al., "Adherence to a Mediterranean Diet and Survival in a Greek Population," *New England Journal of Medicine* 348 (2003): 2599–2608.

2. Demosthenes B. Panagiotakos, PhD, et al., "The Relationship Between Adherence to the Mediterranean Diet and the Severity and Short-Term Prognosis of Acute Coronary Syndromes (ACS): The Greek Study of ACS (The GREECS)," *Nutrition* 22 (2006): 722–30.

3. Luc Dauchet et al., "Fruit and Vegetable Consumption and Risk of Coronary Heart Disease: A Meta-Analysis of Cohort Studies," *Journal of Nutrition* 136 (2006): 2588–93.

4. Thomas L. Halton et al., "Potato and French Fry Consumption and Risk of Type 2 Diabetes in Women," *American Journal of Clinical Nutrition* 83, no. 2 (2006): 284–90.

5. Ramon Estruch et al., "Effects of a Mediterranean-Style Diet on Cardiovascular Risk Factors: A Randomized Trial," *Annals of Internal Medicine* 145 (2006): 1–11.

6. A. A. Alturfan et al., "Consumption of Pistachio Nuts Beneficially Affected Blood Lipids and Total Antioxidant Activity in Rats Fed a High-Cholesterol Diet," *Nutrition, Metabolism and Cardiovascular Disease* 16 (2006): 202–9.

7. Lisa L. Strate, MD, MPH, et al., "Nut, Corn, and Popcorn Consumption and the Incidence of Diverticular Disease," *Journal of the American Medical Association* 300, no. 8 (2008): 907–14.

8. Paul Knekt et al., "Flavonoid Intake and Risk of Chronic Diseases," *American Journal of Clinical Nutrition* 76 (2002): 560–68.

9. B. Wansink et al., "The Sweet Tooth Hypothesis: How Fruit Consumption Relates to Snack Consumption," *Appetite* 47 (2006): 107–10.

10. Dariush Mozaffarian, "Fish, Mercury, Selenium and Cardiovascular Risk: Current Evidence and Unanswered Questions," *Journal of the American Medical Association* 296 (2006): 1885–98.

11. Helen Hermana and M. Hermsdorff, "Fruit and Vegetable Consumption and Proinflammatory Gene Expression from Peripheral Blood Mononuclear Cells in Young Adults: A Translational Study," *Nutrition & Metabolism* 22 (2006): 504–11.

12. Dariush Mozaffarian, MD, MPH, "Cereal, Fruit, and Vegetable Fiber Intake and the Risk of Cardiovascular Disease in Elderly Individuals," *Journal of the American Medical Association* 289 (2003): 1659–66.

13. Lydia A. Bazzano, PhD, et al., "Legume Consumption and Risk of Coronary Heart Disease in U.S. Men and Women: NHANES I Epidemiologic Follow-Up Study," *Archives of Internal Medicine* 161 (2001): 2573–78.

14. Elaine Lanza et al., "High Dry Bean Intake and Reduced Risk of Advanced Colorectal Adenoma Recurrence Among Participants in the Polyp Prevention Trial," *Journal of Nutrition* 136 (2006): 1896–2006.

15. Arja T Erkkilä et al., "Fish Intake Is Associated with a Reduced Progression of Coronary Artery Atherosclerosis in Postmenopausal Women with Coronary Artery Disease," *American Journal of Clinical Nutrition* 80 (2004): 626–32.

16. Alicja Wolk, DMSc, et al., "Long-Term Fatty Fish Consumption and Renal Cell Carcinoma Incidence in Women," *Journal of the American Medical Association* 296 (2006): 1371–76; T. I. Ibiebele et al., "Dietary Pattern in Association with Squamous Cell Carcinoma of the Skin: A Prospective Study," *American Journal of Clinical Nutrition* 85 (2007): 1401–8; Gregory L. Austin et al., "A Diet High in Fruits and Low in Meats Reduces the Risk of Colorectal Adenomas," *Journal of Nutrition* 137 (2007): 999–1004.

17. Martha Clare Morris, ScD, et al., "Fish Consumption and Cognitive Decline with Age in a Large Community Study," *Archives of Neurology* 62 (2005): 1849–53.

18. Marianne Hauge Wennersberg, "Dairy Products and Metabolic Effects in Overweight Men and Women: Results from a 6-mo Intervention Study," *American Journal of Clinical Nutrition* 90 (2009): 960–68.

Chapter 5: Week 5 Goals

1. María-Isabel Covas, MSc, PhD, et al., "The Effect of Polyphenols in Olive Oil on Heart Disease Risk Factors: A Randomized Trial," *Annals of Internal Medicine* 145 (2006): 333–41.

2. D. T. Nash and S. D. Nash, "Grapeseed Oil, a Natural Agent Which Raises Serum HDL Levels," *Journal of the American College of Cardiology* 21 (1993): 318.

3. Ibid.

4. Michael H. Davidson, MD, et al., "Comparison of the Effects of Lean Red Meat vs. Lean White Meat on Serum Lipid Levels Among Free-Living Persons with Hypercholesterolemia: A Long-Term, Randomized Clinical Trial," *Archives of Internal Medicine* 159 (1999): 1331–38.

5. Gregory L. Austin et al., "Diet High in Fruits and Low in Meats Reduces the Risk of Colorectal Adenomas," *Journal of Nutrition* 137 (2007): 999–1004.

6. Eunyoung Cho, ScD, et al., "Red Meat Intake and Risk of Breast Cancer Among Premenopausal Women," *Archives* 166 (2006): 2253–59.

7. Antonia Trichopoulou, MD, et al., "Adherence to a Mediterranean Diet and Survival in a Greek Population," *New England Journal of Medicine* 348 (2003): 2599–2608.

8. Jennifer A. Nettleton et al., "Dietary Flavonoids and Flavonoid—Rich Foods Are Not Associated with Risk of Type 2 Diabetes in Postmenopausal Women," *Journal of Nutrition* 136 (2006): 3039–45.

9. Michelle Micallef et al., "Red Wine Consumption Increases Antioxidant Status and Decreases Oxidative Stress in the Circulation of Both Young and Old Humans," *Nutrition Journal* 6 (2007): 27.

10. Mónica Vázquez-Agell et al., "Inflammatory Markers of Atherosclerosis Are Decreased After Moderate Consumption of Cava (Sparkling Wine) in Men with Low Cardiovascular Risk," *Journal of Nutrition* 137 (2007): 2279–84.

11. Brian Wansink, PhD, et al., "The Sweet Tooth Hypothesis: How Fruit Consumption Relates to Snack Consumption," *Appetite* 47 (2006): 107–10.

12. Kathrin M. Osterholt, MS, et al., "Incorporation of Air into a Snack Food Reduces Energy Intake," *Appetite* 48 (2007): 351–58.

13. M. Macht and D. Dettmer, "Everyday Mood and Emotions After Eating a Chocolate Bar or an Apple," *Appetite* 46 (2006): 332–36.

14. Ka He et al., "Association of Monosodium Glutamate Intake with Overweight in Chinese Adults: The INTERMAP Study," *Obesity* 16, no. 8 (2008): 1875–80.

Chapter 6: Week 6 Goals

1. Rachel N. Close, BS, et al., "The Financial Reality of Overeating," *Journal of the American College of Nutrition* 25, no. 3 (2006): 203–9.

2. Brian Wansink and Pierre Chandon, "Meal Size, Not Body Size, Explains Errors in Estimating the Calorie Content of Meals," *Annals of Internal Medicine* 145 (2006): 326–32.

3. Lene Frost Andersen et al., "Consumption of Coffee Is Associated with Reduced Risk of Death Attributed to Inflammatory and Cardiovascular Diseases in the Iowa Women's Health Study," *American Journal of Clinical Nutrition* 83 (2006): 1039–46.

4. Maria Giuseppina Silletta, MSc, et al., "Coffee Consumption and Risk of Cardiovascular Events After Acute Myocardial Infarction: Results from the GISSI [Gruppo Italiano per lo Studio della Sopravvivenza nell'Infarto miocardico] Prevenzione Trial," *Circulation* 116 (2007): 2944–51.

5. Esther Lopez-Garcia et al., "Changes in Caffeine Intake and Long-Term Weight Change in Men and Women," *American Journal of Clinical Nutrition* 83 (2006): 674–80.

6. Mark A. Pereira, PhD, "Coffee Consumption and Risk of Type 2 Diabetes Mellitus: An 11-Year Prospective Study of 28,812 Postmenopausal Women," *Archives of Internal Medicine* 166 (2006): 1311–16.

7. Jukka Montonen et al., "Consumption of Sweetened Beverages and Intakes of Fructose and Glucose Predict Type 2 Diabetes Occurrence," *Journal of Nutrition* 137 (2007): 1447–54.

8. Lars Libuda et al., "Pattern of Beverage Consumption and Long Term Association with Body-Weight Status in German Adolescents: Results from the DONALD Study," *British Journal of Nutrition* 99 (2008): 1370–79.

9. Sharon Fowler, MPH, et al., Presentation at American Diabetes Association 65th Annual Scientific Session, June 12, 2005.

10. S. Goya Wannamethee et al., "Associations of Vitamin C Status, Fruit and Vegetable Intakes, and Markers of Inflammation and Hemostasis," *American Journal of Clinical Nutrition* 83 (2006): 567–74.

11. Mark Levine, MD, "Criteria and Recommendations for Vitamin C Intake," *Journal of the American Medical Association* 281 (1999): 1415–23.

12. Geraldine McNeil et al., "Effect of Multivitamin and Multimineral Supplementation on Cognitive Function in Men and Women aged 65 Years and Over: A Randomised Controlled Trial," http://www.nutritionj.com/content/6/1/10.

13. Joachim Bleys et al., "Vitamin-Mineral Supplementation and the Progression of Atherosclerosis: A Meta-Analysis of Randomized Controlled Trials," *American Journal of Clinical Nutrition* 84 (2006): 880–87.

14. Scott M. Lippman, MD, et al., "Effect of Selenium and Vitamin E on Risk of Prostate Cancer and Other Cancers: The Selenium and Vitamin E Cancer Prevention Trial (SELECT)," *Journal of the American Medical Association* 301 (2009): E1–E13.

15. G. Bjelakovic et al., "Antioxidant Supplements for Prevention of Mortality in Healthy Participants and Patients with Various Diseases," *Cochrane Database of Systematic Reviews* no. 2, art. no.: CD007176 (2008).

obesity and, 1, 35
risk factors, 119
salt and sodium and, 112
whole grains and, 157–158

Ice cream, 206–207
Ice-Cream Sandwiches, 289
It's Heartly Fare (Harlan), 4

Jams and preserves, 20, 21

Lamb, 196, 219
Lean Cuisine meals, 7, 235, 237, 238, 239, 240
Leftovers, 8, 26
Legumes. *See* Beans and other legumes
Lemons and lemon juice
  Pumpkin-Crusted Trout with Lemon Sauce, 132
  Savory Lemon Rice, 190
Lentils, 30, 31, 164, 165
  Lentil Chili, 32
Lime juice
  Garlic-Lime Flank Steak, 69
  Mojo Pork Tenderloin, 277–278
Liver, 195–196
Lunch
  guidelines on, 25
  making your own, 25–26, 37, 46, 62
  number of calories to consume, 68
  salads, 26, 250
  sandwiches, 22, 25, 26, 37, 62, 251
  serving (portion) sizes, 25, 26, 68
  structure of healthy, 15
  travel and healthy options, 250–251

Maple-Sweetened Collard Greens, 41
Mayonnaise, 26, 186, 211, 252
  Salmon with Caper Mayonnaise, 252
Meal planning, 7–8, 16, 44, 62–63, 131
Meats
  breakfast options, 18
  dinner options, 29, 31, 63
  food labels, understanding, 203
  lunch options, 25
  Mediterranean diet principles, 6, 140, 142, 192–196
  resting after cooking, 60

serving (portion) sizes, 127
types of and healthy options, 84, 192–196
Mediterranean diet
  benefits of, 138, 140–141
  as diabetic diet, 10–11
  principles of, 6, 138, 140–142
  research about, 138, 140–141
  understanding of, 3
  weight loss on, 10
Melba toast, 142
Menu plans
  organization of meal plans and recipes, 7–8
  planning meals, 7–8, 16, 44, 62–63, 131
  understanding food and health eating, 3–4, 5–6, 13
  week 1 goals and menu plan, 15–17
  week 2 goals and menu plan, 59–61
  week 3 goals and menu plan, 97–98, 99
  week 4 goals and menu plan, 137–138, 140
  week 5 goals and menu plan, 183–184
  week 6 goals and menu plan, 221–222, 223
Metabolic syndrome, 151
Milk, 19, 21, 85, 179
Muffins, 20
Mushrooms, 215, 219
  Beef Stroganoff with Egg Noodles, 180–181
  Portobello Burger, 204
Mussels, 171

Nutrition information
  availability of, 2
  food labels, 97, 98, 100–103, 111–112, 181, 203, 211, 215, 235
  nutrition rules, 7
  20/5 rule, 101–102, 108, 158
  understanding of, 2, 59–60
Nuts and seeds
  as healthy fats, 77, 79
  Mediterranean diet principles, 6, 142, 150–152
  nutrition information, 154
  as snacks, 150–151, 212
  umami, 219